ADAM H[

ZERO
PAIN
NOW

–WHAT YOU DON'T KNOW, *WILL* HURT YOU–

ADAM HELLER'S
ZERO PAIN NOW

READ THIS FIRST

The author of this book does not dispense medical advice or prescribe any technique as a form of treatment for medical problems. The intent of the author is to offer information of a general nature to help the reader in their quest to heal psychologically caused physical pain. This book is not to be used as a substitute for a medical diagnosis or medical treatment. If you are experiencing physical pain, you must see a doctor to rule out the possibility of a serious medical illness. All efforts have been made to assure the accuracy of the information contained in this book as of the publication date. The author and the publisher assume no responsibility for any actions of the reader as a result of applying these methods.

...chronic pain costs between $560 billion and $635 billion each year in medical expenses and lost productivity. But, it adds, pain is also personal, affecting each person individually...

— LOS ANGELES TIMES, JUNE 29, 2011
Describing a recent report from the Institute of Medicine, written at the request of the Department of Health and Human Services.

CONTENTS

Since you are reading this book, your pain has already caused you significant disability, distress and money. This book successfully addresses chronic pain, tingling, burning, numbness and other symptoms that are often misdiagnosed and treated symptomatically.

I urge you to experience this profound technique and follow the instructions exactly as written, and you will become pain-free. Adam's technique involves daily action steps both during and after you banish your pain and other symptoms. Do not dismiss this, as the tasks are the key to digging deep and removing the underlying cause of your pain. You've been managing your pain long enough. If I can heal myself using the *Zero Pain Now* Process, you can also heal your own pain. Instead of managing your symptoms, you can finally cure your pain.

Good luck in becoming pain-free.

BORIS BORAZJANI M.D., M.P.H.
Aliso Viejo, CA
July 20, 2011

Anyone can make the simple complicated. Creativity is making the complicated simple.

— CHARLES MINGUS
Jazz Muscian

1

MY TRIUMPH OVER PAIN

It was early 2009 and I was taking my mother to the airport. I picked up her suitcase from the back seat of the car, and felt a huge POP in my lower back. All of a sudden, the scorching pain was unbearable..., I could hardly move. Immediately all the pictures of people I've known with back problems began to flash through my mind. At a supersonic pace, I saw people in traction, people hunched over in pain, people going into and coming out of surgery. I said to myself, Now I've really injured myself. I'm screwed.

Somehow I gathered enough mental and physical strength to get my mother's suitcase on to the curb. I kissed her good-bye, concealing the intense pain I was feeling, and somehow placed myself back in the car. I sat there, rigid, wondering what to do next.

The long day of dealing with excruciating pain was only beginning. My wife's friends from New York were visiting, and they were expecting us to show them around Los Angeles. I was determined to be a tough guy, a real man, and to do whatever I had to do to honor my commitment. I drove home and tried just to get out of the car, but it was as if the pain left me immobilized. I held on to the top of the door and it took me thirty intensely painful seconds to extricate myself from the front seat. I limped slowly into the house...

I explained to my wife, Tamara, what happened. I told her, "I've really hurt myself and I've never felt such severe pain." She immediately said that she would go to Los Angeles alone to meet her friends. She demanded I stay home and rest. Not Mr. Macho. Nobody was going to tell me what to do. I tersely replied, "I'm fine. I can make it. Let's go." After a few minutes of arguing, Tamara realized she wasn't going to sway me, so off we went to Los Angeles. Again, the 30 incredibly painful seconds were spent trying to sit down in the car.

As we were driving, I was secretly hoping that when we arrived at our friend's hotel, we might sit, have coffee, Tamara and her friends could catch up, and then I could head home for a hot bath.

We arrived at the front door of the hotel. Tamara's friends were standing outside. Again, I struggled through the intense pain to get out of the car. Certainly they will see I'm injured and suggest we stay in the hotel, I thought to myself... Wrong!

After the hugs, the first words out of Tamara's friends' mouths were, "Let's go see Beverly Hills." Tamara gave me the glance that said sorry honey. I got back in the car in pain, and off we went to Beverly Hills.

Over the course of the day, this painful scenario was repeated at least ten times. Finally, with our friends safely delivered back to their hotel, we headed home. My entire focus was getting into the house, lying flat on my back, and hoping the pain would somehow go away...

In 1998 my life was a mess. From the outside it looked great. I ran a successful business, was married, and had a beautiful one-year-old son. Everybody was healthy. I had lots of great friends. I had everything most people would hope to have.

However, the external reality concealed a much different internal truth. I felt trapped inside a terrible marriage. I was completely stressed out by my business. I was having panic attacks. My weight had ballooned to two hundred and sixty-two pounds, with an accompanying forty-two inch waist. I developed a terrible case of claustrophobia. I couldn't get into an elevator. I remember checking into a hotel, and the lowest level on which I could get a room was the eleventh floor.

I dragged my bags up eleven flights of stairs. My self-image was battered.

Another time my cell phone was being repaired on the third floor of an office building. When the repair was completed, I was supposed to pick up the phone. When I arrived at the building I walked into the lobby, and froze at the elevator. I pressed the button and when the door opened I reached in, pressed the button for the third floor and immediately stepped out. I watched the floor indicator go from one to two to three, counting how many seconds I would be stuck inside. After fifteen minutes of nervously watching people come and go, I gave up and realized I couldn't get in. Again I needed to devise a plan to cover the embarrassing truth that I couldn't take a simple ride in an elevator. I called the repair shop and told them that I had sprained my ankle that morning playing basketball, and I couldn't walk. It was a total fabrication, the kind I would create regularly to conceal the embarrassment I felt. I asked them to bring the phone to my car. Of course they were happy to be helpful, and a few minutes later my phone was delivered to me. Again my self-esteem had taken a beating.

It wasn't only elevators I feared. I flew regularly for business. The lavatories on jets are very small. I'd sit in my seat really needing to relieve myself and doing everything I could think of to avoid entering the tight, cramped space. Finally when it was absolutely necessary for me, I'd sheepishly enter the lavatory. First I would close and open the door a couple of times to make sure that I knew how to get quickly out. I was petrified that if I moved the latch across to lock the door, it could break and I'd be stuck inside the small space. I'd slowly move the lever over just enough for the Occupied sign to show on the outside of the door, but not far enough for the lever to possibly break. Then my brain kicked into high gear. I began seeing images in my head of getting stuck, of the door not opening, of my losing it and causing a scene. I rushed and got out of there as fast as possible. What seemed like an hour was usually less than two minutes.

I lived sixty-five miles away from my office. Starting in 1995 I began having panic attacks while I was driving. The attacks followed a very specific protocol. On the freeway, when I passed an exit, I would immediately become dizzy. My stomach would churn. My heart would pound and my breathing would become very short and shallow. I felt as though I was going to pass out. The first few times this happened, I was convinced that I was going to die. As I neared the next off ramp all the symptoms would disappear. I had an escape. Then the second I passed the exit - BAM! All the symptoms immediately returned. As the daily panic continued, I could only drive in the right lane so I was closer to the exit. This scenario continued every morning and every evening, three hours each day. By the time I arrived home to my lousy marriage, I was exhausted, stressed and miserable.

My anger was also out of control. My responses to even small inconveniences were disproportionate. On one occasion, I received a call from a customer complaining that the wrong product had been delivered to their location. I hung up the phone and I was incensed. I walked out of the office, entered my car, and slammed the door so hard that my window shattered. This was the first of three times that I slammed doors and destroyed car windows. I was a bubbling cauldron, ready to explode at any moment.

At the time I owned a small airplane. I had begun flying years earlier as a way to get over my fear of flying. Somehow I could get in this small airplane and feel all right, yet while driving my car on the freeway, I'd have panic attacks. Your brain isn't logical. One day I was flying home from a meeting and all at once I was overtaken with panic. It happened so fast. My eyes blurred, my heart felt as though it would pound out of my chest. I was alone, trapped, with nobody to help me. I was sure I was going to die. I did whatever I could do to stay conscious. I was six-thousand feet in the air, terrified, and I didn't know exactly where I was. I was reasonably sure that there was an airport somewhere on my right. I called the air traffic controller and told him that I was feeling ill and needed to land there. He asked me if I needed to declare an emergency. Somehow my ego was still big enough to say no. I asked him to direct me to the runway. Ten minutes later I was safely on the ground and the panic quickly dissipated. My flying days were now over. Another huge blow to my already fragile self-image.

Shortly thereafter, in November, 1998, my first wife and I decided to end our marriage. What was a tumultuous marriage turned into a combative divorce. More stress, more anxiety, more tension, and more fear.

A few weeks after my first wife and I separated, I scheduled a physical with my doctor. I always put examinations off for as long as possible, because I knew that I'd be forced to step on the scale. More bad news I didn't need. However, it had been close to five years since I'd had a physical, so I finally went to the doctor. I used my normal strategy and closed my eyes when I stood on the scale. What I can't see can't hurt me.

The doctor took a blood sample as part of the checkup. When the results came back, there was a problem. My liver enzyme level was very high, almost six times the normal level. My doctor looked me sternly in the eyes and said, "You don't get forever."

That did it. That was all I was willing to take. I decided that now is the time to change. I had many changes to make and no idea how to turn my life around. I just knew I needed to do something.

I decided to start with my physical health. At that point in my life I wasn't yet ready to understand that, as Elmer Green, the famous Mayo Clinic physician states, "Every change in the physiological state is accompanied by an appropriate change in the mental emotional state, conscious or unconscious, and conversely, every change in the mental emotional state, conscious or unconscious, is accompanied by an appropriate change in the physiological state." It really didn't matter where I started, the mind affects the body and the body affects the mind. Weight loss and a healthy liver seemed the most pressing matters, so I chose to focus on solving those problems first.

I visited a local bookstore and began researching how to lose weight and improve my health. I started with a book by Andrew Weil, the Harvard trained medical doctor, and a proponent of integrative medicine. I needed to motivate myself. Since I knew very well how to do the process of fear in my brain, I rallied enough terror to make sure I followed whatever program I chose. I changed my diet, joined a gym, and began to slowly change my beliefs, my behaviors, and create a new life.

After six months of eating well and exercising, my weight dropped considerably and my follow-up blood work showed remarkable improvement. This was my first demonstration of how fast the human body can restore wellness. My impending health disaster was now behind me. I felt that I was gaining leverage over my mind and my body. However, this was only the beginning. I was still struggling every day, with the panic attacks, the fear and the rage. I continued to read everything I could get my hands on about health and wellness.

Then one day I was listening to the Howard Stern radio show and I heard Howard talk about a book on back pain, written by Dr. John Sarno, MD. I'd never had a problem with my back, but I was determined to know everything about becoming and staying healthy. So, I read the book just in case.

I noticed that many of the books I was reading had recommendations on their back covers by Deepak Chopra. I assumed he must know something. I decided to check him out.

I purchased his book entitled *Perfect Health* and began reading. Much of the book resonated with me. Deepak kept mentioning the power of meditation so I decided to learn how to meditate. I went to Chopra's center and was instructed in the process of meditation. This began a spiritual journey that has included many years of daily practice. I eventually became an instructor of a style of meditation called Shakti Pat. I still meditate daily, sometimes for as long as two hours. I love it, yet it did nothing to solve my fears, my phobias, my panic, my runaway emotions and my anguish.

Soon I had read all of Deepak's books. I even took a series of courses and became certified as a trainer by his center. Deepak Chopra is a devoted proponent of Ayurveda, the 5,000 year-old system of health and healing from India. It was 2001, and now that my physical health seemed to be normal, I went to see Deepak's partner, David Simon, for a traditional Ayurvedic physical. I wanted to confirm that my physical health was as good as I believed it was. The experience was enjoyable and I could even hop on the scale with my eyes open!

When the tests were complete, David gave me a clean

bill of health. Though he did notice when he asked me ques-
tions about my ex-wife and my sister, I clenched up like a fist.
He recommended that I read a book by Debbie Ford entitled,
The Dark Side of the Light Chasers.

I quickly read the book and I immediately signed up
for one of Debbie's workshops. This was way out of my box.
Picture this: I'm a left-brained, Jewish, businessman in a big
room with a group of guys hugging each other while Hare
Krishna music played in the background. I remember thinking
to myself, I'm glad nobody I know has any idea that I'm here.

About the same time as I was attending Debbie's
workshop, I made some changes in my business. I was bored
and wanted to shake things up. I owned a janitorial supply
distribution company. It was originally a janitorial service
started by my father Lionel. He built the company into a thriving business. One of the real treats in my life was having the
experience of working with him for twenty years. He was an
amazing man...the most giving, charitable and kind man I've
ever known. He always led by example. He always knew
when someone needed help and he always was there to lend a
hand. We would have lunch together most days. Regardless of
where we ate, people would come to greet him throughout the
meal. In the time we worked together, I only encountered one
person who had something negative to say about Lionel... a
record I'd love to equal. It was during these years that I really
learned from him about the joy and responsibility of helping
others. The more time I spent with my father the more I began

to change my ideas about the purpose of my life. I realized that life isn't all about me. I began to pay more attention to helping others.

One day while thinking about how I could better serve my customers and improve my business, I realized that with my experience in the industry, I could train people how to open and operate their own businesses. As their businesses grew and became more profitable, they would purchase more supplies from me. As they say, a "win-win."

Gibson University was born.

The training was a big success. People started new businesses and began to prosper. Other clients diversified by adding new services and became more successful. At the same time we built strong personal relationships. They eventually began to not only bring their professional problems and obstacles to me, but also their personal problems. I loved helping my clients whom I now considered my friends, move forward towards their dreams. Since I have a Jewish mother, I felt that I could give advice on any subject any time, whether I knew the answer or not--just like mom.

This was the time when the Life Coaching industry was in its infancy. Debbie Ford, from whom I had taken a workshop, began training coaches to do her style of coaching. In addition to learning how to coach others, she promised an opportunity to use the process to make personal changes and create a better life. This sounded like something I needed. I still had the secret fears, phobias and panic.

It was early in 2002 when I began my training. After two years of deep inner work, I grew personally and also earned a certification as a master coach to help others. At the end of the program, my fears were lessened and I felt much better about myself. I was now having great success helping other people make big changes in their lives. I felt incredible joy as my clients flourished. The biggest gain in the program was meeting a beautiful, brilliant coach from Toronto named Tamara. Since I had failed in my earlier marriage, I was certain that wasn't going to happen to me again--ever! I knew that a troubled relationship could wreak havoc throughout my life. You can imagine what happened; one fear I ended up beating in the coaching program was the fear of getting married again. Tamara and I married in 2005, and recently celebrated our sixth wedding anniversary. We are still extremely happy together.

Between 2002 and 2005, as I increased my coaching business, I focused more of my time on my clients and less time managing the janitorial supply business. My coaching clients were having huge breakthroughs and that was incredibly gratifying for me. They were moving through and conquering big problems with divorce, bereavement, weight loss and career problems in a short four month program. I felt exhilarated as I watched my clients create their own positive life changes. My passion had definitely changed from helping people solve business problems to helping them solve personal problems. I decided to sell the janitorial supply business and focus solely on helping people.

By 2005, my coaching career was thriving. Clients were thrilled with their results. I was looking for ways to make improvements. I'm an impatient person and I like to create results faster, so I wondered if there was a way to accelerate results in my own life, as well as the lives of my clients. I was finally feeling like my outer world was in sync with my inner world. I had used every tool and method I learned, to change the way I think. The results of all my hard work was that I was extremely happy. It was a long, gut-wrenching process, but I had been willing to do whatever was necessary to get the results I wanted. I made the changes I needed to make. I was feeling great. However, I still suffered minor symptoms of claustrophobia. It wasn't a huge problem for me, but I was determined to prove that I could solve it and feel even better about myself.

I discovered another method to help clients tackle their issues and improve their lives. It's called Neuro Linguistic Programming (NLP). This is a method created for people to take control of their thinking and make quick positive changes. It's an easy way to understand your thinking, and a rapid way to change your response to anything. After careful research, I decided this would be a very valuable tool to help my clients achieve the results they wanted more quickly than any other technology. Also, the trainers had several techniques that they said would finally help me get rid of my claustrophobia. Off I went for thirty days of very intense training. The techniques were amazing and worked as promised. Instead of attempting to discover why people have problems, the NLP method focuses on how people "do" their problems in their brain, like a recipe for a problem. This was a refreshing and effective way to make positive changes. When you change the recipe in your brain, you get a different result. When you perfect the recipe, you perfect the result - rapidly.

The training was broken into several slightly different sections including NLP, Time Line Therapy™ (another breakthrough method, created by Tad James, to release negative emotions and change limiting decisions and beliefs) and hypnosis. Combined with all the other tools I had already learned and tweaked to get better results, I felt prepared to help just about anyone solve any problem and create a much better life for themselves.

Part of the Time Line Therapy training included what they called a "pain paradigm." This technique was based on the original Dr. Sarno research,[1] and produced much faster results. I remembered reading his book and was very interested in this new process, a very quick method to teach people how to cure their chronic pain. It worked extremely well and was very fast. At the time I wasn't particularly interested in helping people solve their physical pain problems, but I was glad to have another tool to help clients. My goal was to make myself the best agent of change in the world. Every tool that I learned helped me move closer to my goal. Also, while taking the course, I

---

1. Research performed as head of Clinical Rehab, New York University

took advantage and volunteered to be the demonstration client when the phobia technique was taught. Back in the elevators. I wasn't comfortable, but I got inside. Eventually, I created my own technique to help many of my clients successfully and rapidly cure phobias. I used the method on myself and finally healed my own fears. (I'm writing this as I sit in a room on the twenty-seventh floor of a hotel and would not be happy climbing the stairs three or four times each day.)

After two years of study I became a certified trainer of NLP.

Now I was armed with an even broader range of methods for helping clients. I was convinced any physical or emotional problem could be solved very quickly. I spent months combining everything I had learned over the many years of formal training, along with the hundreds of books I'd read about the brain. I was determined and eager to have a way to help people make changes similar to the ones I made, but without the years of tormenting effort. My personal process was grueling. It seemed to me that I could build a practice helping people solve their core issues much more quickly. The result was something I called *Rapid Life Change*, a process that works with any willing client to produce big, positive and rapid changes. Clients got over divorce, the loss of a loved one, phobias, panic, anxiety and a host of other big problems, usually in one intense, five-hour session. The results were astounding. My clients arrived from around the world feeling unhappy, and left feeling great.

As my business grew I began to notice a pattern with clients. As I stated, they came to with big problems. Almost all of them would explain their problems in great detail and then almost as an afterthought, would mention their back or neck hurt, or they had pain somewhere in their body. It appeared that this was much too common to be a coincidence. I remembered what I had learned about physical pain and its psychological causes. In many cases, the pain problem was more debilitating than the original problem they came to solve. The repercussions of their pain created huge limitations. There were the obvious limitations, such as limited mobility. However, their pain had created even greater negative obstacles. There were huge psychological repercussions. Mothers couldn't connect physically with their children by getting on the floor and playing. Not participating in sports kept people from connecting with friends. Socializing was reduced. Drug addictions were common after years of taking narcotics to manage pain. Many clients couldn't earn a living, or, at the very least, the pain resulted in a reduced income. This was in addition to the great financial expense of doctors, drugs, physical therapy and all the other methods for managing pain. When people would share the stories of their pain, they became despondent, even depressed. They were not only hurting physically, they were suffering throughout all areas of their lives.

Intuitively, I knew this was the area in which I would focus and make a major difference. In my earlier studies I had already seen plenty of proof that the cause of most chronic or ongoing pain had a psychological cause. I set out to solve the problem of back and body pain.

First, I used the technique taught in the NLP training. Amazingly, my client's pain usually lessened or completely disappeared very fast. The quick positive results seemed astonishing to me, and as it turned out, a bit too astonishing. After a while it seemed the pain would return. The pain certainly originated in the brain, or the pain never would have disappeared through merely talking about it. Clearly the process needed to be improved to make a pain-free life permanent.

I knew that Dr. Sarno was having long-term success with his patients, even though many required psychotherapy as part of the treatment. It occurred to me that a method could be created that would bring faster results and not require the tedious process of psychotherapy.

I started experimenting with any and every possible combination of techniques. I spent every spare moment in my office for nearly three years experimenting with anybody I met who was suffering from pain. I used the linguistic skills I had been taught to develop a new process that is more persuasive and effective. Small, yet vital changes to the quick technique I learned at the NLP training proved beneficial. Only after having a complete understanding of the underlying cause of pain, and a real change in beliefs, was there a permanent cure.

Finally, after about one hundred successful cases, this process was ready for the public. All the effort yielded a process that I believe will really change the world. This is a way to help you eliminate your suffering and live the life you really want. You can use this method to solve your back pain, neck pain, fibromyalgia, tension and migraine headaches and chronic, recurrent or repetitive pain anywhere in your body. This process works. You can make it work for you. This book is your way to finally and permanently heal your pain.

I finally arrived home from my trip to Los Angeles feeling battered, exhausted and in intense pain. Even with all my history of helping people heal their pain, I had fallen into the same trap as many of my clients. I believed that I had injured my back. It was so obvious. I picked up the suitcase and heard the pop in my back. It must have been a physical injury. It's logical. It's one thing when it happens to my clients, but it's different when it happens to me. All of a sudden, I realized what I had done. My brain had performed flawlessly and diverted my attention by providing pain-searing, intense pain. I said to myself, *I'm the Back Pain Guy.* This entire day was spent in pain so immense that I completely forgot that *I've helped so many people* heal debilitating pain, often much worse than mine.

I locked myself in the bedroom and I began to use the *Zero Pain Now* Process on myself. This is the same technique that so many others have used in exactly the same painful situation. Forty-five minutes later I had successfully cured myself and I was completely pain-free.

Even though I'd witnessed this scenario so many times before with my clients, I now had the personal experience to know that virtually anyone, including you, can heal your devastating and debilitating pain rapidly, without surgery, without drugs, without exercise, and you can start your process, today.

By the way, the next night I was scheduled to play in a softball game. I not only played in the game, I hit my first (okay, my only!) home run of the year.

NOTES

Ultimately I am confident TMS* theory will become part of mainstream medicine for the simple reason it is correct, and more successful at alleviating pain than any other modality..

— DR. MARC SOPHER

(*TMS: Tension Myositis Syndrome, is a term coined by Dr. John Sarno. In Zero Pain Now, we refer to DPS or Diversion Pain Syndrome, as the same condition.)

Back pain is one of the most complicated problems in medicine. It's something I've been working on for 30 years and I still don't understand it.

— DR. JAMES WEINSTEIN

Professor of Evaluative Clinical Sciences & Orthopedic Surgery
Dartmouth Medical School
Los Angeles Times - April 4, 2011

2

HOW TO ASSURE YOUR SUCCESS

Do you believe that the cause of your pain is psychological? This is the question I have asked every client who has
successfully healed their pain with the *Zero Pain Now* Process.
When you are able to answer that question with a bold YES,
you will be well on your way to healing your limiting pain and
moving into a life of freedom from pain.

In 1976, my father, Lionel, was diagnosed with a hernia. He was told that he would need surgery which included a
stay in the local hospital and the usual lengthy recovery. Lionel
was a very smart man. He was determined to educate himself
and look for better options before agreeing to have the surgery.
He knew that just because something had been done one way

for decades, that did not indicate the best, or even an acceptable, method of treatment. Someone told him about a doctor in Long Beach, California, who was using a new procedure to repair hernias. Apparently, the new technique was performed as an outpatient treatment. After the repair, patients would stand up and walk out of the hospital, coming back for a follow-up a few days later. My father asked many of the local doctors about this outpatient option. Every doctor told him this was impossible and a hospital stay was mandatory for the repair to last. Each doctor and surgeon he asked told him This can't work. It will never last. Don't do it. The way we have been doing it for decades is the only proven way...

The amazing success of people using the *Zero Pain Now* Process to heal themselves has exceeded their expectations. This technique allows you to heal yourself. Everybody comes with his or her own story and beliefs system. You may be thinking, "What if I'm the one person the process won't work on?" Although some clients are more resistant, and take a while longer to become free of pain, the process has had total success.

Most people are skeptical that pain can disappear quickly. We are just beginning to realize that how we think, how we use our brain to process and manage emotions, affects us not only mentally, but physically as well. Let's try an experiment: Imagine a lemon. Notice the bright yellow color. Slowly feel the rough yellow peel in your hands. Scratch the peel with your finger and then smell the lemon. Now imagine cutting the lemon in half. See the wet lemon juice glistening. Now imagine taking a big, wet, juicy, sour bite of the lemon. Imagine the sour juice bursting into your mouth. If you are like most people your mouth began to water. All this was going on in your brain and it produced physical changes. This is just one example of how just about every thought you think, changes what you feel. When you think about it, doesn't your pain feel worse when you are focused on it? That's your mind-body connection. When you change the process of what you do in your brain, you change your physical results.

Client after client has shown up in pain, sometimes debilitating pain, and left the office pain-free. Like you, most of these people had serious doubts about how fast this process can work. Sometimes not just doubts, but downright disbeliefs that this process will allow you to finally heal your pain. They believed that they had tried everything to rid themselves of their pain. Maybe you've had a similar experience. They had been diagnosed with some type of structural issue: a bulging disc, a herniated disc, stenosis. Many were told something was affecting a nerve and that was the cause of their pain. Many either had unsuccessful surgeries or were told that surgery was the only option. Other people were diagnosed with fibromyalgia and told to expect a lifetime of drugs to manage their pain. Still others suffered through decades of tension and migraine headaches. Most had already seen doctors, surgeons, physical therapists, acupuncturists, along with many other alternative practitioners. They had taken supplements, done yoga, and all the core strengthening and stretching exercises. Nearly all had spent thousands of dollars, sometimes tens of thousands of dollars, on various pain gadgets and products with the hope that one of these items would finally bring some lasting relief. Every one of these people was searching for some thing, some way, some person, some miracle to help them manage or limit their pain.

In a nutshell, this process offers you the following:

- No surgery
- No drugs
- No physical therapy
- No contraptions
- No aids or gimmicks required
- Permanent
- Fast

It is effective regardless of the location of your pain.

Perhaps you are skeptical about whether reading this book and using the *Zero Pain Now* Process can heal your pain. That's understandable. I want to acknowledge you for continuing to read this book. Perhaps, like most people who have been battling pain, you feel as though you have tried everything and still have discomfort. If you are expecting me to tell you that some structural abnormality is the cause of your pain and you need to rest, take drugs, exercise your stomach muscles, hang upside down on some contraption to lengthen your spine, do anything to treat a structural or spinal problem, or that you are weak-willed, lazy, or not willing to get better, then I must disappoint you. Very rarely have these tactics helped pain sufferers heal your pain. Sometimes they provide some temporary relief. However, as long as professionals continue to place the blame on a structural abnormality, the result will likely be the same short-term pain management.

This method doesn't work that way. At first, you may find some of the things I am about to share with you difficult to believe. However, by the time you finish reading this book, you will change your beliefs about the real cause of your back pain, neck pain, shoulder pain, leg pain, knee pain, foot pain, or the pain anywhere in your body. You will not only understand and believe the real cause of your pain begins psychologically, and then leads to a physical process that produces pain, but you will also wonder how you could have been brainwashed into believing the old-fashioned thinking that anything structural could have been the cause.

The success stories included here are of people with pain similar to you, and they healed their pain after receiving an earlier diagnosis of a structural abnormality by learning and applying the *Zero Pain Now* Process.

The truth is the real cause of your pain starts psychologically and leads to physical pain. The pain is real. It is physical. It can be excruciating to have that physical pain. The good news is that it doesn't start in your spine. Yes, you have probably been given a structural diagnosis. However, if that were true, all the other methods (you've likely tried) would have left you pain-free. If you are open to a new possibility that the real cause of your pain starts with your thinking, and originates in your brain, you will learn something new. This new knowledge will help you comprehend and accept the real cause of your pain. You will see that you can heal your own pain, and feel better. As you read every page of this book, any fear you had that you have to limit your lifestyle will vanish. You will believe that the sooner you resume normal physical activity, the sooner your limitations will disappear, and these limitations will be replaced by a full life. You will understand that when you understand, you will banish your pain.

YOU HAVE NOTHING TO LOSE BUT YOUR PAIN!

This method will assist you in healing your own pain. Your success will come when you understand and accept that the real cause of your pain starts psychologically and leads to physical changes that affect your muscles, tendons, and nerves, and provide you with pain. The knowledge you will acquire as you read, understand, and accept every page of this book will allow you to heal your pain, rapidly.

Again, I'm not a doctor. I'm not a scientist. I'm not a guru. I'm just a guy who worked hard to develop a program that has worked for people who believed their spine, nerves, muscles, tendons or joints were causing them pain. As you follow this program exactly as written, you will take control of your brain and heal your back and body pain. What you don't know WILL hurt you. What you will know, WILL heal you.

So how is it that knowledge is the key to healing your pain when most people with pain have been diagnosed with disc or structural issues? I believe that these diagnoses are incomplete and are based on the false premise that structure or anatomy is responsible for most persistent, recurrent or chronic pain. The real cause is that the pain originates in your brain.

From my remarks you might think I don't like or respect doctors. On the contrary, I have the utmost respect for the medical profession. I think there are doctors who will acknowledge that there are new approaches to looking at old problems. Pain has been around forever and if they are being candid they'll tell you they just don't know exactly its cause.

Almost everybody who has successfully healed their pain using this process has been referred from a doctor. They refer their patients suffering from physical pain, because this method will get you the results that you want. The truth is that most persistent or chronic pain is not a medical issue. It is a psychological issue that leads to physical changes that produce your pain.

If I told you that by following a few simple rules you will be able to become pain-free and resume a normal life, would you be willing to follow these simple rules?

Please say out loud:

"YES, I WILL, FOLLOW THESE RULES, AND, I WILL BECOME PAIN-FREE."

Great.

Now here are the simple rules:

1. **Carefully read every word in this book in order**
2. **Every time you are asked to do something, do it EXACTLY as it is written.**
3. **Do not become pain-free until you can say to yourself, *"I believe the real cause of my pain is psychological."***

If you want to become pain-free and add more freedom and joy to your life, you must choose to change in certain ways. You must choose to learn and to understand something new. You must learn to change how you experience your problem. You must choose how you think. There is always more than one way to look at a problem. When you choose to think differently, you will feel differently. Your act of reading this book will automatically start you thinking in a more useful way. As you are exposed to new ideas about the cause of your pain, your old limiting beliefs and limiting strategies will transform to new powerful beliefs and useful strategies that will produce the results you want. When you choose to understand and accept the real psychological cause of pain, you are, in fact, choosing at this moment to be pain-free.

This process is available to you so that you don't have to endure the short and long-term negative effects of surgery, or ingest potentially dangerous drugs, or hang upside down while stretching on some contraption. You will heal your pain and get back to having the great life you want.

My father did decide to go to Long Beach for the new and better hernia procedure. After the procedure he stood up, albeit painfully, and walked out of the hospital. In a short time he was healed, he resumed all normal physical activities and he was free of pain. He lived another twenty-five years and never had any reoccurrence of a hernia. He was very happy he didn't listen to the old-fashioned medical thinking, and just like you are doing now, he chose to get the benefit of a new, cutting-edge, successful technique.

NOTES

"After 30 minutes on the phone with Adam my pain was decreased by half. 30 minutes later, my pain was gone."

I'd been suffering intense neck pain for months. I believed that I injured myself. I train horses so debilitating neck pain kept me from working. Twice weekly sessions with the chiropractor provided some temporary relief. However, the pain kept returning. One day the pain was so intense that I was stuck in a chair and couldn't move. My wife went to the pharmacy for pain medication.

I had a short and life-altering phone call with Adam. He described Diversion Pain Syndrome, and taught me a simple process. In thirty minutes my pain dropped in half. After the call, I continued the process for another 30 minutes and I completely cured myself. I called my wife and told her I didn't need the drugs.

It's been four years and I'm still pain-free.

— **GREG KALLMEYER**
Horse Trainer
Burlington, KY

When the brain changes, so do we.

— DAVID EAGLEMAN
Author, Incognito

3

HOW WE GOT HERE

When I was a young boy I was a bit chubby. It was a harrowing experience for me to go clothes shopping with my mother and buy the pants labeled "Husky." This took a big toll on my self-image.

My mother adored me and always with the best intentions, would purchase and prepare foods with the aim of helping me lose a few pounds. This made for some of the grossest concoctions. My mother believed that cottage cheese could be substituted for anything, making the dish less caloric and more healthy. I say less tasty and more deadly! She was able to take lasagna, grilled cheese, and her special tuna casserole, substitute cottage cheese for the real thing, and successfully transform the dish into something more suitable to use as an adhesive or a dangerous weapon. One day her creative mind (again, with the best intentions) led her to substitute bean sprouts for spaghetti. She heated the bean sprouts in an early version of the microwave oven to add just the right amount of radiation. Then she poured spaghetti sauce on top. Well, I was a fat kid and was willing to eat just about anything within arm's reach, so I gobbled down the 'beansproutghetti,' A few hours after eating dinner, I had a high fever, nausea, and vomiting. I had the flu. I was down for a few days. However, in my mind, I linked the bean sprouts with illness and vomiting. I couldn't look at bean sprouts for years without breaking into a sweat.

Your brain looks for what is different to link to, and make meaning out of an experience. The first time you ate ice cream, you probably felt wonderful. You linked the good feeling to what was different, eating ice cream, and now you like ice cream. If at the moment you were taking your first bite of ice cream you received a bee sting, your initial linkage to ice cream would be considerably different. You would associate ice cream with pain. This is normally how we form our likes and dislikes. If your early experiences in a car were lovely country drives with the family, followed by a picnic, you are probably relaxed and enjoy being in the car. If your first ride included an accident, followed by a trip to the doctor, you are probably anxious and uncomfortable. This is the way many fears and especially phobias are created in your brain. We unconsciously look for what is different in the experience and then attach meaning.

The point is that the meaning we assign to events and

situations is not necessarily logical, correct or useful. We are just making assumptions, or linkages, that lead to beliefs. When you believe something to be true, you go out and build a world around your beliefs.

As you will learn throughout this book, you can change your beliefs. I've used many of the same techniques that went into this pain relief method for other problems such as my issue with bean sprouts. I was amazed how easily I was able to change my response to just about anything, even bean sprouts. I am pleased to say that I now regularly eat and enjoy them.

In the days before MRI machines and CT scans, doctors used X-rays. If you were to go to your doctor and complain of back pain, you would have probably been told to take aspirin as needed and rest. If your pain persisted, and it was after the year 1865 when Wilhelm Conrad Rontgen invented the X-ray machine, eventually you would be given an X-ray. If the results showed some disc abnormality, you would have been told that must be the cause of your pain. They had a picture that showed something other than what was considered and taught in medical school to be the perfect and healthy spine. The doctor was doing his or her best to help you feel better. The problem was that there was no proof for this diagnosis. It just seemed logical to assume that since your X-ray showed something that looked imperfect, that the abnormality must be the cause of your back pain. Seems logical, right?

In my opinion, that false conclusion has led to the biggest and most costly epidemic facing the Western world today. Reports show that approximately $600 billion dollars is spent in the United States every year, chasing the cure for back pain, or just about any persistent or recurrent body pain. You have surgery. You take dangerous drugs. You are stretched, manipulated and twisted like a pretzel. You try acupuncture. You practice yoga, do stomach exercises, and special core training. You stretch. You swim. You take supplements. You meditate. You take time off work to rest. You spend thousands and thousands of dollars on mattresses designed to conform to your spine. You go to the chains of retail stores or search online to buy all the gadgets, special chairs and devices meant to help you manage your pain... All of this in an attempt to fix an incorrect guess, a hunch not supported by evidence. A conclusion that your pain and discomfort is caused by a structural or disc abnormality. A conclusion that was never the reason for your pain.

Traditional medicine has been unsuccessful in making the correct diagnosis. Perhaps medicine has failed because the problem is not medical, it is psychological. Conventional-thinking practitioners of medicine do not believe that emotions cause physical changes. As Dr. Levin intimated earlier, their lack of mind-body training and time limitations keep most medical doctors from looking at the whole person. Therefore, they are more likely to treat a symptom than the real cause of the problem. The truth is, emotions can and do cause physiological changes in your body. This is why all the treatments and products you have tried have failed to leave you cured and without pain. They are chasing the wrong cause. They are trying to prove that the world is flat.

IF YOUR SPINE WAS THE CAUSE OF YOUR PAIN, THE TACTICS AND TREATMENTS I JUST MENTIONED WOULD HAVE HEALED YOUR PAIN, AND YOU WOULD NOT BE READING THIS BOOK NOW.

Let's fast-forward from the thought processes of 1865 to 1965, exactly one hundred years since the invention of the X-ray. Dr John Sarno M.D. joined the New York University Medical Center, where he is a professor of clinical rehabilitation medicine. His focus involves treating people with back pain, neck pain, shoulder pain, knee pain, etc. His medical training probably taught him the standard protocol - that the cause of pain can be found either in the spine, or is due to arthritis, poor posture, or lack of physical exercise. At that time, the most commonly prescribed treatments for pain were surgery, drugs, heat, traction, exercise and rest. Just like today, those treatments were not very effective in long-term pain relief. As Dr. Sarno wrote in his book, *Healing Back Pain,* "The experience of treating these patients was frustrating and depressing."[2]

Dr. Sarno observed that a staggering 88% of people suffering from pain also had histories of tension and migraine

2 Sarno, John MD, (1991) *Healing Back Pain* p.ix

headaches, hiatal hernia, stomach ulcers, colitis, spastic colon, irritable bowel syndrome, constipation, along with other gastrointestinal ailments. At the time (now confirmed) all of these were considered to be caused by tension. He made the conclusion that this painful disorder affecting your muscles (and now known to affect tendons and nerves) was also caused by tension.

He labeled the disorder "Tension Myositis Syndrome," or TMS. The definition broken out is "myo" for muscle and "sitis" meaning change. Therefore, Tension Myositis Syndrome is a painful disorder caused by tension that causes physical pain in your muscles, nerves and tendons. Through trial and error, Dr. Sarno discovered that the only way to provide lasting change to his patients was through the process of understanding the real cause of your pain.

My own years of study and experience with hundreds of successful clients has indicated to me that a more precise name for the disorder is Diversion Pain Syndrome (DPS). The purpose is to divert your attention from repressed emotions that do not fit inside your self-image, usually anger or rage, to something physical, such as pain.

This updated definition, along with a more streamlined process to expedite long-term healing has enabled 85% of my clients to greatly reduce their pain or become free of pain in a few hours. Over 95% heal themselves within days. Some people take a little longer to heal themselves. However, with persistent use of this method, you will free yourself from your limiting pain.

Just to be clear, not all pain is DPS. There is a difference between acute pain and persistent or recurrent pain. If you break your foot, it hurts. It is supposed to hurt. However, in six weeks your foot has healed. Your body has an amazing way of healing. If the pain is not gone in six weeks, or the pain is recurring at the place of a previous injury, it is probably DPS. There is no such thing as the "old football injury." You may have taken a beating on the field thirty years ago, but once your body has healed, your body has healed.

Keep in mind, Dr. Sarno has treated thousands of patients and reports cure rates of 85 to 90 percent, just using linguistic (only using words, no physical touch) techniques. He has written that most of his patients become pain-free in two to six weeks after his treatment. This was an amazing success.

I consider Dr. Sarno the pioneer in this work. In my opinion, he is the Wright Brothers of curing pain. He made the discovery, he proved the theory, and he treated thousands of people. He believes this process requires the diagnosis of a medical doctor, but I think you'll now agree this is not a "medical" problem.

It occurred to me that if you can heal yourself in six weeks, why not in six hours?

The Zero Pain Now Process was born.

Three additional years of experimenting with various combinations or recipes yielded a specific and unique process that works, and works amazingly well. It is effective regardless of where in your body you experience pain. This is the process of Rapid Linguistic Deconstruction and Repatterning. Put another way, this means rapidly breaking down the psychological and emotional processes that cause your pain, and changing the process to a new way that keeps you pain-free.

As you thoroughly read every word on every page of this book, you will learn and understand the information necessary to heal your pain. Before the end of this book you will understand that most ongoing or recurring pain starts with emotions being repressed. These repressed emotions ignite physical changes in the autonomic nervous system. Blood vessels constrict causing a reduction of blood flow. Blood carries oxygen. Therefore the reduced blood flow results in a slight oxygen deprivation at the effected area. This slight oxygen deprivation produces pain, tingling, burning, numbness and/or weakness. The pain is physical. The pain is intense. The pain is real. The cause of your pain is DPS.

DPS is a process that begins in your brain. It begins as psychological and then turns physical. This process which I call the "Path to Pain" then provides you with a wallop of pain. Understand that the purpose of DPS is to divert your attention from some unbearable emotion, such as anger or rage, to something physical-in your case pain. When you understand and accept the psychology of DPS, you will become pain-free. Thousands of people just like you and me have healed themselves with this knowledge.

DPS Pain Symptoms can show up as:

- Back pain (lower, middle and/or upper)
- Shoulder pain
- Knee pain
- Elbow pain (tennis elbow)
- Foot pain (plantar fasciitis)
- Hamstring pain
- Tendonitis of knee, shoulder or elbow.
- Fibromyalgia
- Hip pain
- Headaches (tension or migraine)
- Whiplash syndrome
- Buttock pain
- Groin pain
- TMJ pain
- Pain in any other areas

You can use the information described here to cure your pain. The word "cure" usually indicates a disease and a medical problem. Your DPS pain is not a disease or medical problem, but you can still cure your pain. As I stated earlier, the problem of most persistent or recurrent pain is not medical. The cause is psychological. The cause is repressed emotions, which starts the Path To Pain. A better term to use than cure, is heal. You will heal your pain with knowledge. When you understand and accept that the cause of your pain is DPS, and you understand the psychology of DPS, you will heal your pain. As Rand said in his success story that you will read shortly, his pain disappeared just like when the flu breaks. All of a sudden your pain will be gone. Does this sound amazing to you? As Walt Disney said, "It's kind of fun to do the impossible."

The truth is that curing your physical pain by changing what you do in your brain only seems implausible, because you have been repeatedly trained to believe that pain starts with some type of an injury.

Everyone I meet believes that his or her pain was caused by some injury. They often demonstrate how they turned or contorted their body to injure themselves. The problem was never with their spine. The problem was in their thinking. As soon as they understood the real cause, and used this approach, their pain was gone. As Dr. Daniel Amen said in his book, *Change Your Brain, Change Your Body*, "When you change your brain, you change your body." This process will help you to change your brain and make a positive change in your body. As long as you follow the three simple rules I described earlier, you will change your brain and heal your pain.

As you can clearly see, the path to your reading these words at this time was a long one. How you got here started before you were born, with the invention of the X-ray machine.

Someone made an honest mistake, albeit a huge mistake, in diagnosing the cause of pain. You have been paying the price since you first felt your pain. You have been paying the price physically, emotionally and financially. That's the bad news.

The good news is that you have made a great choice. You have made the choice to read these words right now. You are choosing to see things differently. Every choice you make matters and the condition of your life is the sum of your choices. Some choices were useful, some choices were not. Some choices are conscious, such as reading this book. Other choices are unconscious, such as the choice to repress "unbearable" emotions, that led you to physical pain.

Every time you read one of my words you are choosing to learn something new. Every time you read a sentence in this book you are choosing to understand that the real cause of your pain is not your spine, but is DPS. As you complete every paragraph you are choosing to believe that you will heal your pain using the *Zero Pain Now* Process. As you continue to thoroughly read every page, every chapter in this book, you choose to become permanently pain-free now.

Lumbar disc herniations are responsible for low back and leg pain in fewer than 3% of cases..

— HL ROSOMOFF, M.D.
Neurosurgeon
Clinical Journal of Pain, 1985

FROM THE CHIROPRACTOR
BY DR. JIM COX, D.C.

Being a skeptic has often prevented me from embracing new ideas. My chiropractic degree was earned at a university that is, for the most part, scientifically based. Accepting a new cure for pain was difficult, particularly for pain that could not be reproduced by administering any orthopedic test. I was taught to perform tests, form a diagnosis based on the results of those tests, and administer an appropriate treatment.

Two years ago, Adam introduced me to the world of Diversion Pain Syndrome and his Zero Pain Now Process. While I do my best to be open-minded, I was not immediately convinced. Where was the scientific evidence?

Many of my patients who come to me in pain have already visited their M.D., or their neurologist, or an orthopedic surgeon, or all of the above. They've had a battery of tests and been given a diagnosis of some structural abnormality, that they are told is the cause of their pain. They've been subjected to therapies and medications, yet their pain remains.

Then they come to me looking for answers. After all, chiropractic is considered alternative medicine, and they hope I will have their answer. As a doctor of chiropractic, I have many tools in my bag of options for such patients, but sometimes I am still at a loss. That was until I started referring patients to

Adam's *Zero Pain Now* Process. Since then, every one of these patients I have referred to Adam has successfully healed their pain, many in one day! Some have taken a little longer, but every patient who has used this process has become free of pain. This is the evidence I was seeking. The evidence is in Adam's results.

My responsibility is great in that I am trusted by the public to do no harm. There must be a trust among colleagues in every healing profession as well, no matter the field in which we specialize. Built on this trust, Adam and I have developed a unique partnership; one I value for its inspiration, education, and above all, service to those who no longer want pain to keep them from enjoying their lives.

DR. JIM COX, D.C.
Laguna Beach, CA
July 15, 2011

Risks Of Medical Errors

7,000
DEATHS FROM MEDICATION ERRORS
IN HOSPITALS;

20,000
DEATHS FROM OTHER ERRORS
IN HOSPITALS;

80,000
DEATHS FROM INFECTIONS ACQUIRED
IN HOSPITALS;

106,000
DEATHS FROM FDA-APPROVED
CORRECTLY PRESCRIBED MEDICINES.

THE TOTAL OF MEDICALLY CAUSED
DEATHS IN THE US EVERY YEAR IS
225,000.

– DR. BARBARA STARFIELD, MD, MPH
The Johns Hopkins School of Hygiene and Public Health
Journal of the American Medical Association
Volume 284, No. 4. 2000

NOTES

4

SUCCESS STORIES

Reading the following success stories is a crucial part of healing your pain. Every story is here to help you become permanently pain-free. This entire book is a process that has been formatted in a specific way. As you will with the rest of this book, please read every word of every success story.

Your *Zero Pain Now* Process begins here. Even if you don't think a story applies to you, please read every word. Doing so will help you permanently rid yourself of pain. A couple of hours reading is a small mental investment to regain a life free of pain, and filled with physical freedom.

My Success Story
Rand Marquardt

I began noticing some slight pain and discomfort in my hamstrings during the summer of 2009. Looking back, I believe I was gradually working my way up to this "dis-ease" over the last four to five years, having gone through a divorce, a change of employment, a lowered income, payment pressures, and perhaps questioning a mid-life crisis about my mortality, and not living up to my personal expectations of success.

I turned fifty on July 4, 2009, when I also noticed some pain and discomfort in my legs and lower glutes. The bottom of one of my feet also felt uncomfortable. I had a more difficult time bending over and running. I noticed I even had difficulty walking normally. My stride was shortened, and I had a hard time keeping up with others. I was always an athlete and a physical education major who prided myself on my fitness and athleticism. I wanted to get back to normal, yet my body wouldn't let me. I woke up stiff and sore in the morning. I knew I had neglected my stretching and yoga; I wondered if this was it, or if I had something else Something wasn't quite right. It was more than just old age sinking in, like everyone was telling me. I knew something bad was going on…

My symptoms worsened going into the fall of 2009, even though I did my stretching and yoga routine, seeking to get my health back. My legs hurt and I was extremely stiff. The discomfort had now spread into my neck and shoulders. I was very uncomfortable and fatigued-more than ever before. I figured it was time to see a doctor; after all, I could justify a complete physical, for having just turned fifty.

I told my medical doctor everything about my body. X-rays revealed a completely normal and healthy spine. My doctor recommended physical therapy. Ouch! You mean *I've neglected my own health that much that I gotta go see some- one else!* While I enjoyed my workouts, I wasn't seeing much improvement, perhaps a ten-to-fifteen-percent gain. I still had this uncomfortable, painful feeling that was spreading through- out my body. I told the doctor it felt like my whole body was experiencing a "pain virus." He discounted my analysis, yet begrudgingly ordered an MRI.

The doctor and I were both shocked when the MRI re- vealed moderately severe to severe blockages in the lower lum- bar (4-5) facet joint. It appeared nerves were inflamed. I felt a full range of negative emotions. I asked myself, Now what?

I was referred to a neurosurgeon. Oh my, I said to my- self, These guys are the brain, neck and spine doctors! At this point I was having a difficult time putting my socks on. Getting in and out of the car was a painful chore. Simple tasks, such as bending to light a fire in the fireplace, or performing even a light workout, were excruciating. It was almost unbearable just to stand up. I walked like a feeble ninety-seven-year-old-man, especially in the mornings. By the afternoon, I was somewhat better able to function.

I was seeing very little benefit from physical therapy. I told the neurosurgeon I was also doing exercises on my own, yet I was getting nowhere. The doctor told me that lower back surgery appeared to be my best option. I was perplexed. I asked how lower back surgery could help with my shoulder and neck pain. How can there be a connection? His answer was, "Pain sometimes shows up in ancillary spots." That made no sense to me. However, I could no longer tolerate this pain, discomfort, stiffness, and lifestyle, any longer. I told the doctor, "Please fix me."

I was terrified of having surgery. The images of being sliced open horrified me. What about all those nerves in the lower back by the spine? I knew that so many things can go wrong in surgery.

I had surgery on December 29, 2009. The surgery was performed by the neurosurgeon. That night I was walking the halls of the hospital on my own, and feeling great. I had the morphine pump handy at all times. I felt really well for the first four or five days upon returning home. Then…the symptoms came back with a vengeance. I was instructed by my doctor to be patient. I still had to wait another four weeks to resume physical therapy.

This time physical therapy was performed using a more "hands on" approach. I loved the personal training and care I received. I was becoming more fit. However, I was still experiencing pain. I revisited my original medical doctor. He prescribed yet another round of physical therapy. I was now diagnosed with fibromyalgia. Oh my God, what is this? I Googled it and found I had most of the symptoms. The future looked bleak. The doctors said, There is no cure.

I was not willing to live the rest of my life like this! I was asking God and the Universe for a way to beat this and cure myself.

I learned that fibromyalgia, along with most chronic or persistent pain, is usually misdiagnosed as structural disc problems. The real cause of the pain is psychological tension and emotion. I didn't know how to heal my pain. I didn't have the correct formula or method. I knew deep inside the problem was psychological, or, as Adam Heller says, "psycho-physical." Yet I kept questioning myself about what the doctors described as my structural problems and fibromyalgia. Could the pain in my legs, feet, lower back, neck, shoulders, and throughout my entire body, have a psychological cause?

At about that time I came across a posting on Facebook from Adam Heller, explaining the *Zero Pain Now* Process. I saw the words "pain-free" and proceeded to read more, and follow up. I had previously heard of Adam. He was well known in the world of self-help. He has a fantastic reputation.

I immediately contacted Adam. He made time to speak with me the same day. I liked what he had to say. I signed up for a session that would begin in a few days; not soon enough for me. I was willing to try anything to get my health back and become pain-free.

Adam began the *Zero Pain Now* Process by sending me a link to watch a video, and to prepare me for our session. Since I lived two thousand miles away from Adam, I had my session using the computer video conferencing software called Skype.

As I began to watch Adam's video I was experiencing intense pain. If I had to rate my pain and discomfort on a scale of one to ten, with one being pain-free and ten being intense pain, I would say most of the time I was between seven and eight. While watching the pre-session video, there were times my pain reached a ten. The searing pain was almost too much to bear. However, as I watched the video, my level of pain began to decrease. By the time I finished watching Adam's *Zero Pain Now* Process video, my level of pain already decreased to a three or four. I was amazed how quickly I was feeling better after just watching Adam's video.

As I went through my session with Adam, the pain continued to disappear. I was feeling better than I had felt in years. The process was so simple, and it was really working. My pain was disappearing without surgery, drugs or physical therapy. We were just talking. This was just as Adam had promised. When I understood that the real cause of my pain was psychological, my pain would disappear. His process was really working.

Our session together was invaluable for several reasons. My pain level decreased, and my understanding of the psychosomatic or psycho-physical cause of my pain gave me enormous peace of mind. I knew I was finally done with surgery and dangerous drugs. I realized that the pain in my neck and shoulders would disappear when I used the *Zero Pain Now* Process. Although some slight pain returned intermittently on occasion, I used Adam's process and the pain went away. This was it! This was the information I needed to finally and permanently heal my pain. For me the *Zero Pain Now* Process was priceless.

About a week later, after our initial session, I e-mailed Adam to tell him that this horrible and painful experience that had taken over my body was completely gone. It was sort of like when the flu breaks. The final bits of pain left that rapidly, and I felt great!

Adam gave me guidance to cure myself, and I am happy to report that I am pain-free and I have the tools and strategy to stay pain-free. I can run, ride my bike, golf, and do every activity that I wish to participate in.

Adam gave me the knowledge and wisdom to take my life back, and the understanding to heal myself. I now have a full and complete life. A life filled with physical activities. I can participate in all the sports I like, and I even have the physical freedom to have a great sex life. That knowledge is really invaluable.

I am most appreciative and grateful for Adam's guidance.

RAND MARQUARDT

Michigan

2011

PSYCHO-PHYSICAL:

A process that begins psychologically, and leads to actual physical changes in the body.

The Chef With The Calf Pain

Janet is a specialty chef at one of the top hotels in the world. She came to me with persistent pain in her calves. Her job involves standing for long periods of time. If she couldn't cure her pain problem, she was in danger of losing her job. Also, she had given up her running, in her words, "the one activity that gives me freedom and energizes me." She asked if I could help her. I've had many successes helping people to heal their back pain, neck pain, shoulder pain, knee pain and foot pain. However, this was my first encounter with pain in someone's calf. In Janet's case the pain was in both calves. I suggested we try my *Zero Pain Now* Process and monitor the results.

I asked her if she would be willing to consider that while her pain was very real, the possibility that the real cause of her pain is psychological. Willingness to fully accept that the real cause of pain is psychological is absolutely necessary.

As Janet told me she was going through a divorce, she immediately grasped the possibility of a psychological cause. We agreed to meet at my office the next day after she was examined by a medical doctor. We began the *Zero Pain Now* Process with my teaching Janet why the real cause of her problem could not be structural. I cited many scientific studies done by major medical centers and very highly regarded doctors and surgeons that prove the cause of your pain is psychological. I explained how the process begins with a repressed emotion, usually anger, or more frequently, rage. I reminded her again and again that this is your brain's way of avoiding the emotion that doesn't fit inside your self-image. When your repressed emotion threatens to erupt into conscious awareness, your brain will provide you with something physical to focus on. In your case the physical result is pain. Sometimes extreme pain. I explained to Janet that the repressed emotion leads to a reduction in the size of your blood vessels. This reduction causes a lessening of blood flow. Blood carries oxygen. Therefore the amount of oxygen is slightly reduced. Usually the reduction is only three to five percent. This slight oxygen deprivation is the real cause of your pain. That's DPS. A slight oxygen deprivation that leads to physical pain, sometimes intense pain. I told her there is nothing wrong with your legs. You have DPS. Since the cause of your pain is DPS, you can heal your pain today.

Janet understood and fully accepted the cause of your pain is psychological. The first and most important part of making it possible for you to heal your pain today is right now to understand and fully accept the real cause of your pain. I explained to Janet that all you need to do to get rid of your pain today is to let your unconscious mind know that you consciously understand the emotion that is being buried.

That's the beauty of the *Zero Pain Now* Process. When your unconscious mind understands that you consciously get the emotion, your pain disappears, usually instantly. Janet and I began the process. As I asked Janet the questions necessary to help her get to her emotion that would make her pain disappear, something incredible occurred. All of a sudden, the pain in both of Janet's calves jumped into her left shoulder. She began holding and rubbing her shoulder. She told me she never experienced pain in her shoulder before; now her calves felt fine and all the pain was in her shoulder. As we continued the process, five minutes later the pain suddenly moved again. This time the pain went to Janet's lower back. If there was any question about the DPS pain having a non-structural psychological cause, that question is now answered. All of a sudden Janet's body and posture changed. She said, "The pain is gone. Completely gone," with a big smile. Janet was astounded.

She bent over, stretched, contorted her body in different positions and there was no pain. Janet healed her pain. The total time it took Janet to get rid of her pain was one hour and twenty-five minutes. This is a very common result. Janet left my office thrilled. I occasionally see her running around the hotel where she works with a big smile on her face. You can have the same great results as Janet when you understand and accept the real cause of your pain.

Surgeons must be very careful
When they take the knife!
Underneath their fine incisions
stirs the culprit - Life!

— EMILY DICKINSON
Famous American Poet

The Golfer with Low Back Pain

Larry loved to play golf. He played three times per week, with his usual foursome, at his local country club. He also traveled throughout Europe playing many of the old famous courses.

About fifteen years ago, Larry began to experience pain and stiffness in his lower back. It seemed to become worse after each round of golf. Larry was told by his club professional that lower back pain is common among golfers. He said, "The pain is a result of a swing that is not smooth." Larry took many golf lessons from the pro, hoping his improved swing would cure his pain.

Over time, Larry's pain began to worsen. He decided to visit a chiropractor for an evaluation. The chiropractor gave Larry an adjustment and recommended rest. In a couple of weeks Larry's back was feeling better, so he went back to the country club to play golf. That evening Larry's back began hurting again. He continued to play golf. He developed a regime to lessen the pain so he could continue to play. He stretched for twenty minutes before each round. On bad days Larry would swim for thirty minutes before stretching. He was doing whatever he could to loosen his back.

As time progressed, the pain continued to get worse. Sometimes the pain would move from his left side to his right side. Occasionally Larry's pain would shoot down one of his legs. Also, sitting in a chair for too long began to cause him pain. Sitting for the long flights to Europe became even more painful.

Larry's pain finally became too much of a problem. He went to visit his doctor. His doctor prescribed an MRI.

When Larry received the results of his MRI, he was devastated. The image showed a bulging disc in his lower back. His doctor told him that this was the cause of his pain. The doctor recommended surgery to repair his spine.

Needless to say, Larry was not happy. He was a very successful executive. His "A"-type personality did not allow for anything or anyone other than him to control what he needed to do.

Larry began doing research. Since he was a perfectionist, he did his research very well. He searched online for other alternatives to surgery. He asked everyone he knew about other methods of relieving his pain.

Eventually, Larry was chatting with a doctor who has referred people to me to help them heal their pain. He sent him to see me. Larry was feeling desperate and he was willing to go in a new direction. Since traditional pain management methods were not helping Larry with his back pain, he called me to inquire about a session.

I explained to Larry that my experience has shown that most persistent pain does not have a structural cause... the cause is usually psychological. I explained that the pain is real. The pain is physical. However, the cause usually begins in your brain. I cited major studies that show two out of every three people who have never had pain have bulging discs or herniated discs.

Larry was intrigued. I told him that in order for me to help him heal his pain, he would have to answer an honest "yes" to one question. I asked Larry "Are you open to the possibility that the cause of your pain is psychological? He answered with a resounding, "Yes."

We scheduled his session for the following Monday. After taking a history of his pain, Larry and I began the session. As always, I began with almost an hour of teaching him about the real cause of his pain. This part of the process is invaluable, because the cure is understanding and accepting that the process of back pain begins in your brain. I quoted all the studies that have concluded that structure rarely is the cause of pain. I taught him that what I call the Path to Pain begins psychologically, with buried emotions. These buried emotions begin a physical process where your blood vessels constrict. This results in slightly less blood flow. Blood carries oxygen. Therefore, the real cause of most persistent pain is a slight oxygen deprivation. I continued to teach Larry about DPS pain, and how his thoughts have everything to do with his lower back pain.

After about an hour, Larry completely understood and accepted the psychology of DPS. He understood that DPS pain is the brain's way of diverting your attention from "unbearable" psychological emotions to something else...in Larry's case--lower back pain.

This information and some follow-up assignments would have been enough for Larry to heal his pain. Enough isn't good enough for me. It was at this point that we added the final exercise in the Process.

As we began the final exercise, Larry's level of pain was a very painful eight out of a possible ten. This is the process utilized that assures approximately eighty-five percent of my clients become completely pain-free, in less than an hour. After ten minutes, I checked with Larry, and his level of pain had dropped to a three. Always a great sign, because any change up or down in the level of pain is more proof that the cause of pain is psychological. All we were doing was talking. Talking does not change your spine. Therefore if uncovering buried emotions changes your level of pain, your spine has nothing to do with your pain.

I continued the exercise with Larry. After another ten minutes, I again checked on Larry's level of pain. It had increased to a five. This is common. Sometimes as you get close to the buried emotion that is causing your pain, your brain will turn up the pain as a last attempt to distract you from the buried emotions.

As we continued, Larry stopped answering my questions. He began to tell me that he remembered an event years earlier that occurred at work. His largest client had left his company and given the business to one of Larry's ex-employees. Even though Larry was furious and filled with rage that his client would "screw him," he knew there was nothing he could do about the situation. In his words, he "toughened up and went forward." This was the first time Larry recognized the rage he was carrying for all those years. I asked him when this incident happened. He answered, "1994." I said to Larry, "Interesting, that is about the same time your lower back pain started." I noticed Larry's physiology changing. His shoulders appeared more relaxed, and his breathing appeared to slow down. Once again I asked him his level of discomfort. He gave me a half smile and said, "Almost zero. Maybe one half."

I ended the session. I gave Larry some mandatory tasks to complete. I told him to do them and send me daily updates as to his progress.

Since Larry is a perfectionist and very dependable, he performed the tasks perfectly. On the third day, Larry sent me an e-mail that stated, I played thirty-six holes of golf today and I am pain-free. I didn't believe it possible. It works.

Drugs are not always necessary. Belief in recovery always is.

— NORMAN COUSINS
Journalist

The Entrepreneur Who Found The *Zero Pain Now* Process

Alex had been in pain on and off for most of his life. His first attack of pain occurred when he was sixteen years old. The year was 1986 and he was traveling in Vienna. Seemingly out of nowhere he was struck with excruciating back spasms. He immediately sought medical care. The doctors recommended rest so he was confined to bed for a week. This initial bout of pain lasted only a couple of weeks. However, Alex has suffered occasional back-muscle spasms since that first incident.

On September, 8, 1999, Alex suffered what appeared to be a back injury. He was moving some equipment. He heard something in his back. All of a sudden, his lower back was in intense pain. In addition to the back pain, Alex had pain running down his right leg.

Upon investigation, the doctors diagnosed Alex with a disc bulge. They told him that was the cause of his pain. His doctor recommended surgery to correct the disc. Alex just wanted to make the pain disappear, so he agreed to have the surgery.

Alex's surgery appeared to be a success. He was feeling better. Except for the on-and-off muscle spasms, he was again mobile and able to function.

In 2005, Alex's back went out again. He again had pain in his lower back. This time the lower back pain was accompanied by shooting pain down his left leg. Again the doctors diagnosed Alex with a disc bulge. Again the problem was the very same disc that led to his last surgery. Here he was again. The doctors again recommended surgery... another laminectomy. Alex was disheartened. However, always the good patient, Alex again agreed to have the surgery.

After the surgery was completed, Alex began his recovery. This time his recovery was much more difficult. He was taking much longer to feel better. However, Alex is a perfectionist. He doesn't let anything stop him from reaching his goals, so he persevered.

Shortly after his recovery from his second surgery, Alex began to experience pain in his neck. The pain also was shooting down both of his arms. In our session he described to me that his neck would just tense up. He began to see chiropractors to "adjust him." This offered him some temporary relief. After each visit to the chiropractor, approximately two weeks later his pain would lessen.

Over time, Alex continued to suffer pain. In addition, his range of motion became more limited. Even when writing, his hands would "tense up" and he would feel pain.

Finally, Alex called me and asked me to help him. I asked Alex to watch my video in his home to begin his healing process. A few days later, Alex arrived at my office for his session.

We began his process with my asking Alex about the history of his pain. I asked him what was going on in his life when he experienced his first back pain. He told me that he had just left his family at age sixteen, and had to be on his own. He indicated this was a very stressful time for him.

I then asked him about his life experiences, and when the next major back pain surfaced. He told me he was in the midst of a very unhappy marriage. His emotions were tattered. However, always putting his best face forward, nobody knew what was going on inside Alex.

When I began to ask Alex about the next major back pain problem, he immediately cut me off, and told me at that time his business was very successful. He was making "a lot of money." He was going out to the clubs at night and working very hard during the day. He was feeling a great deal of stress trying to hold together his lifestyle.

As you can see, there is a pattern in Alex's history of pain. Every time he had a major attack of pain, there was a great deal of stress in his life. Alex was a perfectionist, and he had a strong need to be liked by others. Therefore, he didn't want anyone to see what was going on inside him. He repressed his "unbearable" emotions and went about his life. Eventually, when those emotions threatened to erupt into his awareness, he was blasted with a dose of DPS pain.

Unfortunately, Alex's pain was attributed to disc abnormalities that led to unnecessary and unproductive surgeries.

As always, I continued our session together by explaining to Alex that the real cause of his pain was DPS. I showed him many studies that prove disc abnormalities rarely cause pain. Alex is very smart. He was willing to understand that the cause of his pain originated in his brain. The real case was psychological. DPS begins with buried emotions that lead to a real physical change. The result of the physical change is usually pain. He knew the pain was physical.

When Alex fully understood and accepted that the cause of his pain was psychological, he was ready to heal himself from a lifetime of pain.

We began the final exercise. Alex understood that when he was able to make conscious the emotion(s) he was repressing, his pain would disappear.

In about forty-five minutes, Alex's pain began to lessen. Each time we took a short break I would ask him his level of pain. It moved down from a three, to a two, to a one, and finally, zero. Alex had banished his pain. When he understood the real cause of his pain, Alex was able to make himself pain-free. I've seen Alex several times. I am pleased to report he is still free of his old limiting pain.

If you get (start) to believe something really, really strongly, it can fire up and reach every cell in your body and transform your body.

— CANDACE PERT, PH.D.
Pharmacologist from Johns Hopkins School of Medicine,
Author, "Molecules of Emotion."

Source: YouTube, Miraculous Healing 2 of 2

The Retired Basketball Player With The Bulging Disc

Matt had a successful career as a basketball player. His situation was typical. He began playing ball as a young boy. As he started to excel, he spent more of his time playing ball. He starred in high school and college. He was always one of the best players on his team.

After college, Matt wanted to play professional basketball. While he was an amazing basketball player, he was unsure whether or not he was good enough to play in the National Basketball Association, the best league in the world. He received an invitation to play professional ball in Europe.

Matt considered his options. His dream was to be an NBA star. However, he had a sure thing in Europe. Matt loved new challenges, and decided to opt for Europe. He packed his bags and left.

Shortly after he began playing with his new team, Matt began having lower-back pain. He was a tough guy. Nothing was going to stop him. So he continued to play through the pain.

As his pain became worse, Matt developed ways to manage his pain. He took over-the-counter medication. He stretched for hours. He tried physical therapy, a chiropractic,

Nothing is more fatal to health than over care of it.

— BEN FRANKLIN

and acupuncture - all the standard ways to deal with back pain.

Matt continued to play and play well. He was very determined and very dependable. Matt had a strong need to be liked and he knew that if he played well, people would like him. Once he warmed up, his pain seemed to disappear. Shortly after he finished playing, the pain would return. He knew that when his basketball career was over, when his daily abuse of his body ended, so would his pain.

Matt continued this way for six years. Younger and stronger players arrived. Matt was now an "old man" of twenty-eight, so he retired.

Unfortunately, even though Matt was no longer pounding his body, his lower back continued to hurt. His pain seemed to even become worse. Along with his regular lower-back pain, sometimes he experienced pain in his neck.

Matt finally decided that something must be wrong. He went to see a doctor. After testing Matt to determine that he had nothing organically wrong with him, such as cancer, the doctor recommended an MRI.

Matt was startled by the results of the MRI. He had a disc protrusion (herniated disc). He was told by his doctor that surgery was his best option.

Matt was desperate to avoid surgery. As he said, "The thought of having no control, while being sliced open on an operating table was more than I could bear." So Matt continued to seek other advice. He consulted with two additional doctors. Both gave him the same advice. They told him that surgery was his best option. Matt felt as if he had no choice. He called his doctor and scheduled the surgery.

Three weeks later, Matt had surgery. The recovery went well. He was diligent in following his after-care program. His pain was gone. He was pleased that his problem with back pain was behind him.

Five months after Matt's surgery, he received an approval from his doctor to begin playing basketball. He was told to take it slowly. Matt began playing on a regular basis. He slowly increased his level of play. One morning when he awoke, he felt some discomfort in his lower back. Nothing major, but he was concerned. Throughout the day, Matt's pain became worse. That night the pain was too much for him to sleep. He was afraid he had done some something to re-injure himself.

The next day he went to see his doctor. Once again an MRI was recommended. The results came back showing another problem with the very same disc that had "caused" Matt's earlier pain. Matt was upset. He was again told that he should consider surgery.

Matt decided he was not going the surgical route again. He would find another solution. A better solution. A friend of

Matt's had been a client of mine. He recommended that Matt speak with me. Matt called me the next day.

We spoke on the phone for about thirty minutes. I explained to Matt about DPS and that it starts psychologically and then leads to physical pain. Matt's history of pain seemed like DPS to me. I told Matt that since he was already being treated by a doctor, that I would need a referral to help him. He requested a referral from his medical doctor. Matt was told that the MRI showed proof of a structural problem with his disc. Matt was adamant about wanting to try the *Zero Pain Now* Process. He finally persuaded his doctor to provide a referral to me.

I asked Matt to watch my video before coming to see me for our session. As he watched the video, he began to feel different. Something very unusual was happening in his body. As he was learning about the cause of his pain, his pain was lessening. He was experiencing immediate relief.

Matt's session was scheduled for the following week. When Matt arrived, he told me that his level of pain had fluctuated from very little pain to extreme pain, over the last few days. He learned, while watching my video, about the psychological cause of most persistent or chronic pain. When the pain became worse, he began to focus on his emotions, and his level of pain decreased. Every time. Matt was amazed. He now absolutely knew that his pain could not be structural, because he had some control over the level of this pain just by what he did in his head.

Knowledge is the real power in curing DPS pain. When my clients understand and accept the real cause of their pain, it's usually easy for them to heal their pain.

I spent about an hour with Matt, teaching him about the real cause of his pain. I explained that the Path to Pain begins psychologically by repressing your emotions. This leads to actual physical changes that produce the pain. The pain is very real. It just isn't caused by anything structural.

Matt asked about the time he had broken his ankle, at age twelve. I explained the difference between acute pain and persistent pain. When you break your ankle, it hurts. It's supposed to hurt. Six weeks later your ankle is healed. Your body has an amazing way of healing itself from a real injury. Anytime pain lasts more than six weeks, I suspect DPS is the culprit.

Matt understood and accepted the information I gave him. His pain was still at a level of five out of ten. We began the final exercise. This is the portion of the process when about eighty-five percent of my clients completely heal their pain. The aim of the process is to identify the emotion(s) that began the Path to Pain. Normally, as soon as you identify the emotion(s), the pain disappears.

As I began the exercise with Matt, his level of pain began to increase. He looked more uncomfortable. I asked him his level of discomfort and he told me that it was "now at a seven." As we continued, Matt's pain became worse. It was now at a nine. He was visibly in pain. I explained to him that this is not uncommon. Sometimes when you get close to uncovering the source of your pain, the pain can escalate. This is even more proof that the cause of pain is not a disc.

All of a sudden, Matt's posture changed. I asked him what emotion he was feeling and he said, "Anger." He then told me how angry he was at himself for choosing to play basketball in Europe instead of trying to play in the NBA. He then said, "I'm absolutely filled with rage that I gave up the chance at my dream life." I asked Matt about his level of discomfort. He stopped, flashed me the smile that says everything and said, "Nothing. Nothing. The pain is gone."

As soon as Matt uncovered the buried emotion that was the cause of all his years of lower-back pain, his pain disappeared. Matt was amazed and he was very happy.

I gave Matt some mandatory follow-up exercises to make sure he stayed free of pain. He had healed himself by changing the way he thinks. When he stopped burying his negative emotions, there was nothing to start his Path to Pain. I told him that if he were to go back to his old strategy of burying his emotions, that his pain would probably return. As long as he performed the mandatory follow-up exercises, he would permanently change the process of how he deals with his emotions, and he would stay free of his pain.

As I do with every client, I gave Matt my cell phone number. I told him if he experienced any pain, to immediately stop, and use the information that he learned to banish his pain. Any future pain would only be a reminder that he was burying emotions. I told him that if he was in pain, and needed me, to call my cell phone.

I am pleased to say that I did receive one call from Matt. He called me about seven months after our session. He was playing basketball three or four times per week. He has experienced slight pain a couple of times. As soon as he stopped and used the technique that he learned, the pain disappeared. He had experienced no pain for the last four months. He just wanted to call me and say, "My life is fantastic."

I learned a long time ago that minor surgery is when they do the operation on someone else, not you.

— BILL WALTON
NBA Basketball Star

The Meditation Teacher with Intense Pain

Cindy had every personality trait of someone who would probably experience DPS pain. She was very spiritual, a do gooder, a perfectionist, a people pleaser and had a strong need to be liked. Most of her non-working hours were spent either teaching meditation or performing some service to help other people. Many spiritual people have labeled many emotions as "bad." Experiencing anger or rage isn't okay to most spiritual people. They are all about the love.

Cindy is also a perfectionist. She is incredibly dependable. Her upper-management position for a large company requires that she be very organized and efficient. She is both. Even to the point of being a bit compulsive. According to Cindy, there is a correct place for everything. Every dish, glass and utensil in her home is organized by size, type, color and use.

So far I have described three of the personality traits that seem to show up in people with DPS pain. Cindy also adds a fourth common trait: she has a strong need to be liked. Cindy always shows a big smile, has a hug for everybody, and always over delivers both in business and in her personal life.
Cindy was working out at the gym one day (remember, she is a perfectionist, so she also needs to be in great shape), when she went from bending down to standing up, she felt a pop in her

knee. At first Cindy felt slight pain in her knee. However, later that night, Cindy's knee pain was severe. She rested for a few days. Unfortunately, her knee did not improve.

Cindy went to see her doctor, who ordered an X-ray. The pictures showed nothing structural. She was sent home for some rest. The rest was to be followed by physical therapy. This is a standard medical treatment.

After completing ninety days of physical therapy, Cindy's knee pain had not improved. Her doctor was one of the growing number of medical practitioners who understands the benefits of alternative therapies. He recommended that Cindy try acupuncture. Cindy immediately made an appointment, and began regular treatments. After another ninety days, no improvement.

Cindy returned to her doctor, who now ordered an MRI. To Cindy's surprise, the MRI results showed a structural abnormality. Cindy consulted with two orthopedic surgeons. Both recommended surgery. Cindy hated the idea of surgery, but she wanted the pain to go away. Cindy had her knee surgery three weeks later.

Cindy's recovery after surgery went smoothly. She went through physical therapy. In a short time, Cindy was back to her normal routine.

Four months after Cindy's knee surgery, she began to

experience back pain. Cindy was flabbergasted, and frustrated. She had just been through almost a year of pain management, surgery and recovery. Now she had pain in a new area of her body.

Cindy's first attempt to get rid of her pain was a visit to a chiropractor. She made a great choice. After telling the chiropractor about all her knee problems and now her new back pain, she received a surprising diagnosis. The chiropractor was familiar with DPS. He had referred several of his patients who he was unable to help alleviate their pain to me in the past. He knew that very often, after surgery, people with DPS pain often experience pain in "new" areas of their body. He checked Cindy and diagnosed her with DPS. He then referred her to me for a session.

We began the session with the usual hour of my teaching Cindy about the real cause of her pain. I told her about DPS and that the purpose of DPS is to divert your attention from repressed, "dangerous" emotions, such as anger or rage, to something physical, like pain. Since the purpose of DPS is to divert your attention from your buried emotions to physical pain, surgery has one of two common outcomes. Sometimes the pain comes back to the same area. This is usually blamed on scar tissue. Or, as in this case, you develop pain in a new area of your body. Surgery was only working on a symptom, not on the cause of the pain. Therefore, since the purpose of DPS is to divert your attention from the emotions to something physical, the pain has to return somewhere.

Cindy understood the psychology of DPS. She understood what was really going on in her body. She now believed the cause of her pain was DPS and the cure is understanding and accepting the DPS theory. She quickly grasped that by focusing on the emotions, she can make herself pain-free. She understood that once she consciously understands the buried emotion, there is nothing from which to divert your attention. That is when the pain disappears. Cindy got it.

We began the final exercise. In about five minutes, Cindy stopped the process. She said to me, "My pain is gone." Cindy needed no more than to begin focusing on psychological emotions. Once she did, her pain disappeared. Most people need to uncover the exact buried emotion that is causing the pain. Not Cindy. Once she began to think psychologically, her pain was gone.

I told Cindy that she must perform the mandatory tasks for the next thirty days. She changed how she thinks and her pain was gone. We discussed that if she went back to her old style of thinking, her old strategy of repressing emotions, her pain would return.

Cindy agreed. She performed her mandatory tasks every day. She sent me daily updates, not only describing to me that she performed her tasks, but also writting about her physical activities, none of which resulted in any pain.

In the sick room, ten cents worth of human understanding equals ten dollars worth of medical science.

— MARTIN H. FISCHER, M.D.

The Mother With Back Pain

Laura was the mother of three beautiful children. She called me and told me about the years she had been suffering through back pain. She told me that she was always able to "tough it out." She indicated that nobody would ever suspect that she was in pain. However, Laura had been through enough suffering, and asked me to help her end her battle with pain.

After agreeing to see Laura, I asked her to watch a pre-session video at her home before coming to my office for her session. We scheduled her session for the following week.

When Laura arrived at my office for her session, she said, "Your *Zero Pain Now* Process video really resonated with me." She had a background in psychology, and understood the psychology of DPS. Understanding and accepting the real cause of pain is essential to eliminating the pain.

Since watching the video, Laura had already begun thinking psychologically about her pain. She was surprised that her level of pain had already decreased. She wondered how that could be possible, since she had not uncovered any specific emotion(s). I explained to her that everyone is different. Some people will become pain-free by simply focusing on the psychological process instead of the physical pain. Other people need to uncover the exact emotion(s) to banish their pain. A few need to feel the emotion to free themselves of pain.

We began the session. I asked her about the history of her pain. She told me that the pain first started approximately twelve years earlier. She was in an automobile accident. She was diagnosed with whiplash. She visited a chiropractor. The results were negligible. Interestingly, this was also around the time she began studying for a doctoral degree, and it also coincided with the birth of her first child. As she was telling me this, she instantly linked the stressful time in her life with the beginning of her pain.

Her pain continued intermittently over the years. The whiplash never completely healed. Usually, she experienced a dull pain. She was able to manage the pain. She developed enough rituals to manage her pain and continue with a full life.

About nine years later, she had another attack of intense pain. This was the same time Laura was about to defend her doctoral dissertation. A clear pattern was becoming apparent. When Laura was going through stressful times in her life, she experienced more pain. This is very common with DPS pain. Almost always, the more intense pain occurs when something stressful is going on in your life.

Laura understood what I was saying. She clearly saw the link between the level of her pain and the stress in her life. Not only did she understand, but she also completely accepted that the cause of her pain was DPS. She now believed that her pain began psychologically. She understood that the process then creates physical changes that provide pain. Sometimes searing pain. Laura also knew that she would be able to heal her pain. She had already witnessed her level of pain decrease after only watching my video.

When we started the final exercise, something unusual happened. The final exercise is the part of the process that assists people in pain to become pain-free almost immediately. The exercise is designed to quickly uncover the buried negative emotions that start the Path to Pain. Some of my clients have been temporarily resistant, and unwilling to make conscious their buried emotions. When I asked Laura about her emotions, she would respond with "Happy" or "Joy." I hunkered down, expecting a long process. However, after about five minutes, I asked Laura on a scale of one to ten, what was her level of discomfort. She closed her eyes for a few seconds and answered "Zero."

Of course Laura was happy. In five minutes, she healed twelve years of pain. She was already free of pain before the exercise even began! Simply understanding and accepting that the real cause of her pain was not structural, that it was not whiplash, that it had nothing to do with her automobile accident, was enough for her to end her battle with pain.

I have spent many years helping people learn how to heal their back pain and return to a full life. Most people are successful and free of pain before they leave my office. Usually, the entire process takes a couple of hours. Laura had partially healed herself before she even came in for her session.

Since most persistent or chronic body pain is not a medical issue, but a psychological problem, understanding is the real cure.

Laura demonstrated how quickly you can heal your pain using my *Zero Pain Now* Process. I don't heal anyone. When you grasp and completely accept the DPS theory, you will abolish your own pain.

The Old Football Injury That Wasn't

Phillip had been suffering from back pain for almost forty years. He played football when he was in high school. In eleventh grade, during a practice, he was blocking another, much larger player. Phillip was trying to move the other player, when he twisted his body in an unusual way. He was immediately struck with severe pain in his back.

The coach removed Phillip from the game. After a few days suffering with continuing pain, his mother brought him to the family doctor. Phillip had X-rays taken. The results showed no structural problem in his back. He was instructed to rest, and told that the pain would eventually go away.

After a few painful weeks, Phillip's back was completely healed. He resumed his participation with the football team. Occasionally, usually after a hard practice or game, Phillip would experience minor pain. He was told that he was aggravating his earlier injury. Phillip believed that the end of his football career would be the end of his pain. Until then, he would continue to tough it out.

Phillip eventually graduated from high school and left for college. He was now an ex-football player. Once he arrived at college, Phillip began playing tennis. He was a good athlete. After a couple of years, he was good enough at tennis to play on the school team. Phillip was a bit of a perfectionist. He practiced more than any other player on the team. He regularly stayed after practice to hone his skills. Phillip believed that if he was going to do something, he was going to do it well.

After a few months playing with the tennis team, Phillip's back again began to hurt. He thought that his injury had healed. He had been pain-free for over two years. Phillip was tough. He did not intend to let the pain stop him from being a great tennis player. His coach told him that his old football injury was acting up. He would just have to live with the back pain.

Phillip created rituals to manage his pain. When he warmed up, the level of pain decreased. He stretched for long periods of time. He also took aspirin on a daily basis. Phillip continued his routine of pain management through the rest of his time at college.

When Phillip graduated, he took a job at a large investment firm in New York. Being a great athlete, Phillip was always recruited to play on the company softball and basketball teams. He invariably participated with much gusto, always aiming to be the best at whatever he did.

Unfortunately, there was a cost to Phillip's tenacity. The more he played, the more his back hurt. He sought medical care. He was told by doctors that his old football injury was probably going to hamper him for life. But there were no radiographic findings. He was told by his doctors that this was something he was going to have to live with.

As the years went along, the pattern of trying to manage his pain continued. Stretching and aspirin helped reduce the pain. New alternative methods of treating pain became popular. Phillip went to a chiropractor. This treatment helped for short periods of time. Then acupuncture became the "hot new thing." This did nothing to help him feel better. Phillip did all the exercises to strengthen his core. He was in great physical shape. However, his back still hurt when he was active and when he played sports.

Eventually his pain became debilitating, and Phillip completely stopped participating in sports. He focused his attention on his career, and his family, and he became very successful. Phillip remained the perfectionist he had always been, and he was very dependable. Eventually, he started his own investment firm and became extremely wealthy.

Phillip's life was consumed by his career. He worked fifty or sixty hours every week. The rest of his time was spent with his family. Even though he was not participating in athletics, his back continued to hurt. He was doing nothing to aggravate his old injury, yet he was still experiencing pain. His back didn't hurt all the time. As he says, "But when it hurt, it really hurt." The pain was limiting Phillip's ability to live a full life and he was willing to do anything to feel better.

Eventually, Phillip's search for help led him to a very knowledgeable and open-minded doctor. This doctor was familiar with DPS and the *Zero Pain Now* Process. The doctor suspected that I could help, and Phillip was referred to me.

Phillip and I spoke on the telephone for about twenty minutes. He told me about his old football injury. He believed this was the cause of his lifetime of pain. I told Phillip that in my experience, there was no such thing as an old football injury. In my experience, the human body is a magnificent healing machine. According to Daryl Rosenbaum MD, "As a general rule of thumb, we sort of pick four weeks as the general range for most fractures to heal." While speaking to Phillip about his life of pain, he also told me that he had suffered from bouts of heartburn on-and-off for most of his adult life. I knew that 88% of people who suffer from DPS pain also have a history of some gastrointestinal problems. Stress and tension contribute to, or cause, both.

Phillip met all the criteria for DPS. We scheduled his session for the next week. I asked Phillip to watch my video and to do some homework that included making lists of anything in his life that produced stress, tension or anger. Always the perfectionist, Phillip performed the tasks and brought his lists typed and perfectly organized.

Phillip's session was typical. I spent the first part of the session teaching Phillip about the real cause of his pain. I went into all the details, showing that his pain had a psychological cause. Yes, the pain was real. However, the process that led to his pain began in his brain. I showed him all the professional studies that prove structural problems rarely cause persistent or repetitive pain. Within an hour, Phillip was a believer. He not only understood the psychology of DPS, he also believed that the origin of his pain started in his brain.

Phillip was ready to finally rid himself of his lifetime of pain. He knew that he was the only person who had the power eliminate his own pain, to become pain-free at last.

Now Phillip was ready for the final exercise in the process. Phillip understood that his pain began with buried emotion(s). He knew that when he identified the emotion(s) that were causing his Path to Pain, that his back pain would disappear.

I asked Phillip on a scale of one to ten, what was his current level of discomfort. He replied with "four." As we continued the exercise, Phillip's pain level fluctuated. It went down to a one, then up to a six. As we continued, Phillip uncovered a great deal of rage. There were various events in his life that he had completely forgotten, yet when we were doing the exercise, he remembered these events and felt his rage. I noticed Phillip's physiology change. As he was telling me about a specific situation that produced anger, his entire body began to relax. I asked him his level of discomfort, and he said,"No pain." Just that fast, his pain was gone.

The purpose of DPS is to divert your attention from what your unconscious mind considers to be unbearable emotions, such as anger, or rage, to something physical, like pain.

When you uncover the buried or repressed emotion(s) that are the cause of your pain, there is nothing from which to divert your attention. At that moment, the pain just vanishes. That's what happened to Phillip. He uncovered the emotion and his pain was gone. After forty years of suffering, his back pain was gone.

I gave Phillip some mandatory exercises to follow-up with at home. Of course he performed them with his normal perfection.

It has been two years since I last heard from Phillip. I am told by a common friend that he is still happily free of pain.

Do You Believe The Cause Of Your Pain Is Psychological?

NOTES

5

CHANGE YOUR BELIEFS
CHANGE YOUR STRATEGIES
CHANGE YOUR WORLD

There are a myriad number of teachers who teach programs on leadership. They say things like, I want to train new leaders to go out and change the world. Unfortunately, many of these teachers train their students just enough to lead them back for more trainings. They say they want to train leaders. However, what they really want, are followers.

The sole purpose of this book is to simulate my very successful one-on-one sessions, and provide you with the information so that you understand how... you will lead yourself out

"*I used the process to heal my pain and lose 40 pounds.*"

Adam's *Zero Pain Now* Process helped me heal both physically and emotionally. After one session with Adam, I was finally willing, and able to return to all physical activities. Not only was I free of any pain, the side benefit was that since I was able to get back in the gym, I lost 40 pounds!

I left Adam's office feeling jazzed about living again. I learned about Diversion Pain Syndrome, and a technique to easily change how I manage my emotions, so I can remain free of physical and emotional pain, forever.

It's been four years and I'm still pain-free.

— **CHERYL SMITH**
Publicist
El Segundo, CA

of pain. Since understanding and accepting the psychology of DPS is the way you will say good-bye to your pain, that is the proof your problem originates in your brain. Since knowledge is the cure, the cause must be psychological.

The words in this chapter will offer you so much more than just helping you rid yourself of physical pain. Your beliefs and your strategies determine the world you live in. As always, as you are reading this book, pay very close attention while you continue to read this chapter. This lesson is of great value to you in your rapid quest to banish your pain. When you really understand the power you have to change your beliefs and change your strategies, you have the wherewithal to create the life of your choosing.

All problems are the result of flawed beliefs and strategies. Yes, every problem you have arises from your beliefs and strategies. You will see that as you now change your beliefs about your pain, you will become pain-free. As you choose to change your old limiting beliefs from, I believed that structural issues were the cause of my pain, or, I believed my disc problem was the source of my pain, or, I believed stenosis was the reason for my pain, or, I believed fibromyalgia was permanent and I was stuck with my pain, to your new powerful beliefs such as, I believe that the real cause of my pain begins psychologically with repressed emotions and leads to a physical change that produces pain, or, I believe that with every word I read in this book I move closer to banishing my pain, or I believe I will use all the available information in this book to heal my pain, you will heal your pain. As industrialist Henry Ford said, "If you believe you can do something, or you believe you can't do something, you're right."

Let's begin with one of the great misunderstandings on the planet. People believe their beliefs are true. Yes, your beliefs are your truth. However, they are not true. Beliefs are ideas that you reinforce over a period of time until you believe them to be true. Sometimes this period of time is one second, other times you take years to choose to accept a new belief.

Let's explore the evolution of a belief. This example has nothing to do with political preferences. Some years back Barack Obama decided to run for President of the United States. When he made his announcement, very few people believed he could win the election. One of his opponents was Hillary Clinton. She was a powerful force and very well known. The initial polls showed that Senator Clinton had a very large lead. As the Primaries began, Obama showed some good results. He surprised many people when he won the Iowa Caucus, a major primary. When he beat Senator Clinton in Iowa, more people began to believe that Obama could win. At this point in time, most people still believed that Obama would lose. As time moved along and the Primaries continued, Obama continued to chip away at Hillary Clinton's lead. Eventually, he did beat Senator Clinton. He then beat John McCain in the general election, and became President of the United States. Unless you have just awakened from a Rip Van Winkle sleep, I suspect that you now believe that Barack Obama would win the race and become President. At some point between February 10, 2007, the day Obama announced he would run for President, and November 4, 2008, the day he won the election, you changed your beliefs about his becoming President. As you can see, your beliefs change.

I remember a few years ago I believed that eating tomatoes was a healthy choice. One day in 2008, someone died and some health official blamed the death on his eating tomatoes. According to the official, salmonella from a tomato was the cause of death. In one quick moment I had a new belief. I believe that eating tomatoes is dangerous. Then the officials changed their message. The salmonella is not in the tomatoes, it's in jalapeno peppers. OK, another belief change. Now I believe eating tomatoes is healthy and I believe eating jalapeno peppers is unhealthy. Beliefs change. Not many years ago I believed that I will never get married again! I met an amazing woman. We dated for a year. Now I believe I am a happily married man. My beliefs and your beliefs change.

Are you beginning to see how this works? You change beliefs all the time. At least once in your life, you probably had the belief that someone was the perfect partner for you and you will be happy together forever. Are you still together with that person you were madly in love with in middle school or high school? Take a moment and think of one or two of the thousands of beliefs you have changed over your life.

All the beliefs I've mentioned so far were changed by

outside situations. In his book, *Virus Of The Mind*, Richard Brodie states, "The only way we learn and grow is by changing our belief systems." What if you decide to change any beliefs you have that are not giving you the results you want, into a new powerful belief that will get you the results you want?

Yes, you can consciously change your beliefs to optimize your life. How will your life be different when you transform your old beliefs about the cause of your pain to new and more useful beliefs? Choose right now to say, "I believe the cause of my pain is DPS. I believe DPS starts with repressed emotions such as anger and rage and creates a physical change that is the cause of my pain. I believe that the purpose of DPS is to divert my attention from psychological emotions to something physical, like pain. I believe that since the purpose of DPS is to divert my attention from "unbearable" emotions like anger, and rage, that when I am consciously aware of the repressed emotion, there will be nothing for DPS to divert, and my pain will be gone."

The most important step in changing your beliefs is making the decision to change, now. In the past, your unconscious mind has made the decision for you. Like the examples I stated earlier, something happened outside and you now have a new beliefs. Richard Bandler, the co-creator of Neuro Linguistic Programming, often says, "Control your brain or your brain will control you." When you decide to take control of your brain, you can change any beliefs and create a new reality for yourself. A reality that does not include your old limiting pain.

Strategies, on the other hand, are like recipes. A strategy is a series of mostly internal representations, usually pictures, sounds and feelings, that leads to a predictable result. These strategies usually operate out of your awareness at the unconscious level. We all run these strategies before we do anything. In an extreme example, someone with a phobia of spiders will run a strategy that leaves him or her with intense fear. I had a client one time who had an overwhelming phobia of spiders. I first asked him some questions to uncover the strategy he was using to produce the fear. I asked him what he did in his head just before he was afraid. He said, "I see a picture of a six-foot hairy spider hiding around the corner." Then I say to myself, "He's going to attack me." Then I'm afraid.

If that was what I was running in my head, I'd also be afraid of spiders. My client never forgot to run that strategy when he was coming upon a corner. The corner was the trigger and in less than a second, he had intense fear. The result was very predictable. A corner, the strategy and then fear.

A strategy is a process you run in your head before you do anything. You have a motivation strategy, a decision strategy, a buying strategy, a strategy to know when to feel loved and when to be attracted to someone. You run a strategy before you do anything. Most of the time your strategies provide useful results. For example, when you woke up this morning did you enter the bathroom and put the toothbrush in your ear? Probably not. You didn't consciously do anything. However, your strategy resulted in your placing the toothbrush in your mouth.

This is the result of a strategy that works well.

Anytime you have a behavior that is not giving you the results you want, or is giving you the results you want, it is the result of a strategy.

Much like beliefs, you can choose to change a strategy. By changing any part of a strategy, you will change the result. When you make the correct change, you will get the results you want.

If you were going to bake a chocolate cake, you would need flour, sugar, milk, chocolate, eggs, etc. If you were to take the chocolate out of the recipe and replace it with strawberry, what would happen? You would now have a strawberry cake. When you make any change in the recipe, you change the result. Strategies work the same way as recipes. When the phobic replaced the picture of the six-foot spider with a picture of a little tiny spider the size of a lady bug, his fear didn't appear. A little change can make a huge result. Stanford Psychology Professor Carol Dweck wrote in her book titled, *Mindset*, "Even the simplest change can have a profound impact on your life."

I once worked with a professional figure skater. Her mother died after a long battle with cancer a year earlier. Every time she thought of her mother she felt sad. She asked me to help her solve the problem. Just like you, she wanted to feel good. After a few questions, she uncovered that every time she thought of her mother, her strategy began with an image of her mother just before she died. As you can imagine, the image was not particularly attractive. If that was the unconscious image I ran every time I thought of a loved one, I would also be miserable. So we did a very short process so she could consciously change the image of her mother to an image that made her smile. We practiced linking the new positive image of her mother each time she remembers her mother. That was all that was necessary to solve her problem. We tested the new strategy and when she thinks of her mother she now feels wonderful.

So to recap: A strategy is a series of mostly internal representations, usually pictures, sounds and feelings, that lead to a predictable result. How does this affect you? Because your pain is really the result of a flawed strategy. You have been running a strategy that resulted in repressed negative emotions, such as anger or rage. As you become aware that was what you used to do, you can change the old strategy to a new strategy that focuses on your emotions. The purpose of DPS is to divert your attention from your emotions to physical pain or other symptoms. When you now begin to think psychologically and focus on the emotions, you will become pain-free. That's a useful strategy.

Beliefs and strategies are the filters through which we create our reality. Perception is reality. Your beliefs and your strategies create your perception. Therefore, when you change your beliefs and strategies you change your reality.

As you continue to read and understand this information, you are learning. Learning how to change. Changing how you think. Thinking about the process. Processing the new and useful information you are learning.

Banishing your pain using this *Zero Pain Now* Process requires you to adopt some new beliefs and change some old strategies.

Believe that the cause of your pain is DPS. Believe that the purpose of DPS is to divert your attention from psychological emotions to physical pain. Use your new strategy to focus on your emotions. Consciously run your strategy over and over until it becomes your new, automatic way of thinking.

You be your own leader. Use your new knowledge to create everything you want in your life. Believe you can, and you can... banish your pain and have a full and active life of curiosity, fun and enjoyment. Lead yourself wherever you want to go.

Do You Believe The Cause Of Your Pain Is Psychological?

There is no question that the things we think have a tremendous effect upon our bodies. If we can change our thinking, the body frequently heals itself.

— C. EVERETT KOOP, M.D.
former U.S. Surgeon General

My Success Story
By Kate Hughes

When I was a young child, I asked my father what happens to someone who doesn't wash their hands after using the bathroom. He replied, "They die." Mom taught me never to sit on a toilet that wasn't ours. I was never allowed to let my face touch a hotel pillow.

At the same time my brother was abusing me. He beat me, sat on my head, and pulled my hair. He knew I was allergic to smoke, so he sat next to me and blew smoke in my face. He also sexually assaulted me.

My mother was aware of these intolerable acts, but said there was nothing she could do to stop the behavior.

I just accepted it.

This started a forty-year battle with germs. I just wanted to be clean again. My life was completely limited. I even washed bread after I noticed a piece touch the bag. Every time I returned home I needed to shower and change clothes. I kept hand sanitizer throughout the house.

My freedom was completely gone. I was a slave to a perceived threat. It was bad enough that my life was so limited, but now I was inadvertently teaching my young children to behave the same way.

Then the headaches began. These weren't ordinary headaches. These were knock-down, drag-out, debilitating headaches. It felt like someone took an ice pick and suddenly slammed it into my skull. My only option was to grab my head, scream, and fall to the floor. Sometimes they only lasted ten minutes. Other times the searing pain continued for several hours. The pain was horrendous. I felt as though my head were full of habanero peppers. Just when I thought the pain couldn't get any worse, it did. I couldn't hear, see, or feel anything other than the immobilizing pain.

Every medical doctor I visited tried different drugs. Each had very limited success and brought a multitude of side effects. I tried therapists for the obsessive disorder, but received little benefit. They simply tried to get me to do things that were uncomfortable. Their drugs also didn't cure me.

I needed to do something--anything. I wanted to change for me and, more importantly, I needed to get better for my kids.

I prayed and prayed for help.

Shortly thereafter the family was together for Christmas. My sister-in-law kept praising Adam and the process he used with her to lose weight. She had one session with him and she no longer had any desire to eat junk food. She actually changed what foods she liked and disliked in her brain, in just a few hours with Adam. She was genuinely happy, and free from her issues with food. She said I could use Adam's process to help myself too.

I called Adam and asked if he could help me with my fear of germs. He was really positive and made me feel very safe, so I decided to have a session with Adam. He sent me some easy tasks to do for a couple of weeks before my session. He promised that these tasks would help me get better quickly.

Finally, the day came for our session. I didn't know what to expect. There was laughing, tears, surprises, and more laughing. After the session, my life began to change. Every day I was doing things that would have been impossible for me to do before. I began going out more. I played with and enjoyed my kids. People were noticing the new me. My husband was thrilled!

Now that the germ problem was solved, it was time for Adam to use the *Zero Pain Now* Process to help me with the horrible headaches. We had one session, about two hours long. Adam taught me about Diversion Pain Syndrome. I learned that the process started with repressed emotions. Then Adam asked me some simple questions to help me identify the emotions. Everything changed for the better. It was so sudden. Almost all the headaches stopped. Every once in a while when I start to feel a little pain, I use this as a reminder to focus on my emotions, and I quickly rid myself of any pain.

Thanks to Adam and his process I was able to heal myself. I got my life back. My kids have their mom back. My husband got his wife back. This process was literally the answer to my prayers.

Doctors at Hadassah Hospital in Jerusalem reported finding no difference in the incidence of low back pain in people with or without osteoarthritis of the spine.

— HADASSAH HOSPITAL
Source: Healing Back Pain (DVD)
Mumbleypeg Productions, Inc.

NOTES

6

UNDERSTANDING DPS

What if the only thing you need to do to banish your pain, regardless of how long you've battled your pain, is to read and fully understand this chapter? What if understanding and accepting the words you will read in this chapter are all you will need to permanently rid yourself of pain? It is effective regardless of the location of your pain.

Would that be useful to you? Would that be worth a little time? That's worth a little effort, isn't it? Wouldn't a little concentration and focus, to make a huge positive change in your life, be a great idea? Since understanding the real cause of your pain is the way to permanently heal your pain, this chapter is the key to your freedom. Freedom from pain. Freedom from suffering. Free yourself from the limitations of the limiting beliefs and misunderstandings that have kept you from the full life that's possible for you. NOW... is the time for you to decide to open up to a new understanding and heal your pain with your personal *Zero Pain Now* Process!

Thousands of people with similar problems to yours and mine have understood and accepted that the real cause of your pain is Diversion Pain Syndrome. When they understood and fully accepted the DPS diagnosis, their pain disappeared. No surgery, no drugs and no physical therapy. These are people just like us. Some suffered in pain for decades. Their lives were smaller and more limited due to their back pain or neck pain or their persistent pain. They had given up running, jumping and moving freely. Some stopped traveling or going out. Playing with the kids and grandkids was torture and/or was given up completely. Many enjoyable activities were preceded by a long complex list of rituals to try to limit and get through the harassing pain...or the activities were entirely discontinued. People developed all sorts of complex strategies to deal with, and manage their pain. They saw all the doctors, chiropractors, acupuncturists, and homeopaths. They'd done yoga, physical therapy, taken all the supplements. Just like you, they thought they had tried everything to manage their pain.

Instead of just managing your pain, you have the opportunity today to permanently banish your limiting pain. Understanding the DPS process has helped thousands of people heal their pain. It worked for them and it will work for you. You will feel the freedom that will be yours when all the limitations that came with your pain disappear. When you learn and completely accept that the real cause of your pain is DPS, just like all those before you, your pain will disappear. Knowledge is the real "magic pill" to make your pain disappear. Understanding and accepting the words you are reading in this chapter is that knowledge.

Diversion Pain Syndrome is a change in blood flow to muscles, nerves and/or tendons caused by tension. The tension is the result of repressed emotions. The emotions are repressed because they are not aligned with your self-image. These emotions are considered too terrible and dangerous by your unconscious mind. Therefore, your unconscious mind represses these "dangerous" emotions. This repression begins a process that produces pain and other symptoms. DPS is a harmless or benign condition that affects your muscles, nerves and tendons. DPS can cause pain, sometimes very intense pain. Common symptoms also include burning, tingling, numbness and/or weakness anywhere throughout your body. This *Zero Pain Now* Process has helped people just like you, with DPS, conquer pain in their backs, shoulders, elbows, knees, calves, feet, groins, heads, and virtually any other areas of the body.

The beautiful quality of DPS is that you can completely heal yourself rapidly through understanding. Many of you will have either greatly reduced your level of pain or will be completely free of your old pain before you finish reading this book.

The big myth is that the cause of pain is structural. That herniated discs cause pain. That bulging discs cause pain. That lifting is bad for you or moving is bad for you because it creates structural problems. Some preach that strong stomach muscles are the key. The truth is that almost never do structural abnormalities cause pain. I will demonstrate the validity of the prior statement repeatedly throughout this book. As long as you continue to focus on your body's structure, you will continue to have pain. Almost never (and by almost never I mean approximately three percent of the time) do structural issues have anything to do with pain. Millions of people, perhaps just like you, have been given incorrect diagnoses.

Most medical professionals tell their patients that their pain is attributable to a structural abnormality. Most common is any abnormality that can show up on an MRI, X-ray or CT scan. The pain is blamed on a long list of possible culprits. This list includes:

1. Bulging disc
2. Disc protrusions/extrusions "herniated disc"
3. Narrowing of the spine
4. Bone spurs
5. Spinal stenosis
6. Scoliosis
7. Torn meniscus
8. Osteoarthritis
9. TMJ
10. Normal aging, and other conditions

My experience with many clients has shown that these conditions rarely cause pain. The real cause of most pain is Diversion Pain Syndrome.

So what is DPS? DPS is a psycho-physical process. The "Path to Pain" starts psychologically and produces a physical result. In your case the physical result is pain, tingling, burning, numbness, weakness or all the above.

A proper definition is that DPS is a psychogenic and psychosomatic disorder. "Psychogenic" simply means a physical condition, such as pain, that originates in your brain or is changed by your brain to serve a psychological purpose. It appears to be physical but the real cause is psychological. "Psychosomatic" is a subcategory of "psychogenic" and indicates an actual physical change takes place. In your case the physical change occurs in your muscles, tendons and/or nerves. I prefer to use the term "psycho-physical" because many people have attached or "anchored" negative meaning to the word "psychosomatic." People frequently ask me, "Are you saying the pain is in my head?"..."Are you saying I'm mental?" The answer is the pain is absolutely not in your head. You are not mental. You are perfectly normal.

DPS exists as a defense mechanism. The sole purpose of DPS is for your brain, more specifically your unconscious mind, to divert your attention from the psychological to the physical. More precisely the purpose of DPS is to divert your attention from what your unconscious mind considers to be unbearable emotions, to more acceptable physical issues. In your case, pain is more acceptable than the unbearable emotion(s) of anger or rage. Anger and rage are the most common repressed emotions resulting in pain. Of course the repression of other emotions can be the cause as well. This is critical for you to... understand this now. The purpose of DPS is to divert your attention from what are considered to be dangerous emotions. Emotions such as anger, rage, fear, sadness, shame or many others.

According to your illogical unconscious mind, you would rather be doubled over in pain than deal with these "horrible" emotions. Therefore your unconscious mind provides you with an attack of DPS to divert your attention from the emotion(s) to something physical. In your case the physical result is pain. Of course your conscious mind knows you would much rather acknowledge the negative emotion, immediately become pain-free and go out and have a full life. However, your unconscious mind works much differently. It is your unconscious strategy of avoiding these negative emotions that has kept you in pain.

We all regularly experience psycho-physical occurrences. Here are some examples: My teenage son loves to hide behind a door and just as I am entering the room, he jumps out and yells boo. Of course, I jump back and for a few moments my heart beats much faster. My blood pressure rises and I breathe much differently...but he hasn't touched me. His action has triggered a psycho-physical occurrence. My process starts psychologically and leads to physical changes. Just before I speak to a large group I feel some anxiety: perhaps "butterflies" in my stomach and a little dry mouth. Another common psycho-physical process. Whenever you are startled by a loud noise or have a "near miss" while driving, you experience psycho-physical results. How about turbulence when flying? How does your body react to that psychological trigger? This physical response to a psychological cause is a normal and very regular occurrence. In the case of your DPS, the psycho-physical result is pain.

When you understand and completely accept the psychology of DPS, your pain will disappear. I see it happen every day. Clients come into my office, suffering with debilitating pain, and they leave pain-free.

This method is not magic, hocus-pocus or mind-over-matter. It is a simple process of understanding and accepting the psychology of DPS. DPS is a harmless condition that sometimes produces unbearable physical results.

You have a self image. A way you see yourself and want others to see you. Perhaps you see yourself as a good parent, successful, dependable, smart, in control, spiritual or a good person. When your emotions aren't congruent with your self image, your unconscious mind represses the emotion. This is an everyday simple coping mechanism. For example, if you consider yourself to be a good, loving mother or father, and you have a chronically sick child, it probably is not okay for you to be angry and filled with rage at having to take care of your child. However, it is almost impossible not to have some anger or rage in such a situation. So what you do is push down or repress the anger and rage, and go about your day. You deal with whatever you need to deal with. Or how about taking care of a sick parent? You tell yourself, they did everything for me and now how can I be angry at having to take care of them? Repress the emotion and go on. Perhaps at work you have a boss (or client) that treats you miserably. They expect the impossible from you. Do you scream at them and jump up and down? No. You probably consciously grit your teeth and smile, but unconsciously you repress the emotion and do your job. What about when someone cuts you off while driving on the freeway? Most of us simply push down the anger, maybe let out a quick four-letter word and keep driving. It is this method of contending with difficulties that leads to the cause of your pain. Remember the purpose of DPS is to divert your attention from psychological emotions to something physical. In your case, pain.

Imagine you have a balloon. Every time you bury an emotion it's like blowing a little air into the balloon. Your spouse said something your didn't like--a little blow into the balloon. You look in the mirror and don't like what you see--a little more air in the balloon. You are struggling to pay your bills--more air in the balloon. Health problems--more air in the balloon. Can't find your car keys--more air in the balloon. Your cell phone isn't working--blow. Can't get online--blow. Traffic--blow. Anyone with a family, with a job, with a life, has many occasions every day to add more air to your balloon. Every blow is an emotion that is not OK for you. Therefore, you bury the emotion and continue to move forward with your life. Your unconscious process or strategy is to bury these "awful" emotions. Your process has always been to blow air into the balloon. You are making deposits and no withdrawals. So what happens when the balloon has so much air and the emotions are about to burst into awareness? You get pain. When your unbearable emotions threaten to burst into awareness, you get pain. Sometimes your pain can sneak up slowly. Other times your brain will give you a DPS wallop while you are participating in some physical activity. Remember, the purpose of DPS is to divert your attention from psychological emotions to something physical. In your case, the physical result is pain.

If you have DPS there is nothing structurally wrong with your back, or your neck, or your shoulder, or any other part of your body. DPS only exists to distract your attention away from the psychological emotions to the physical pain. Therefore, when you understand and fully accept the psychology of DPS, your pain will vanish. Focusing on your physical pain is like the glue that keeps you in pain. When you focus on the emotions instead of the physical pain, your pain will disappear. When you become conscious of the buried emotions, you have defeated the entire purpose of DPS, because there is nothing left from which to divert your attention. When there are no buried emotions, there is no pain. You can permanently say goodbye to your limiting pain.

The repression of your emotions begins to construct a physical path that I call your "Path to Pain." It's a pain strategy. Your Path to Pain is a psycho-physical activity that begins with unbearable emotions buried in your unconscious mind. As I have already stated, these are emotions that don't fit your self image, how you want to be seen in the world. This is a simple coping mechanism that all of us use on a daily basis. Expressing your rage every time something negative happens in your life would probably not be very useful and would not give you the results you want. So what do you do? You push it down and go about your life. You repress anger or rage and go on with your day. Your buried emotions stay neatly tucked away, out of your awareness. However, when your unbearable emotions threaten to burst into your conscious awareness, your Path to Pain continues.

The second step in your Path to Pain is a change in your autonomic nervous system. Your autonomic nervous system is a subsystem of your central nervous system. This subsystem operates unconsciously, out of your awareness, performing many tasks to keep your body functioning and healthy. One of the tasks of your autonomic nervous system is to control blood flow. So the initial change on your Path to Pain is a slight constriction and narrowing in the size of your blood vessels. Simply stated, your blood vessels get a little smaller. This result of the smaller opening for blood is a slight restriction of blood flow. Blood carries oxygen. Therefore, with the restriction in blood flow comes a slight oxygen deprivation. This slight oxygen deprivation is the final step in causing your pain,

PATH TO PAIN

Psycho-Physical Activity

Unbearable Emotions
Buried in Unconscious Mind

Change in Autonomic
Nervous System

Reduction of Blood Flow

Oxygen Deprivation
at Effected Location

RESULT

- Muscle Pain
- Nerve Pain
- Tendon Pain
- Numbness
- Tingling
- Weakness

tingling, burning, numbness and/or weakness.

The cause of your DPS pain was never structural. discs never were the cause. The purpose of DPS is to divert your attention from your psychological emotions to something physical, like pain.

When you focus on your physical pain you can't focus on the real cause of your pain: repressed emotions.

When you focus on the psychological emotions that cause your pain instead of focusing on the physical pain, you will be on your way to a permanent cure.

It is only this slight deprivation of oxygen that is the real cause of your pain. Have you ever applied heat to your affected area and had some temporary relief? Your pain eased for a little while. Did the heat change your spine? No. Did the heat repair your discs? No. Heat increases blood flow. Increased blood flow brings more oxygen. That's why your pain decreases for a short time. That's why DPS is a benign process. There is nothing structurally wrong. It's just less oxygen at the point of your pain. When you have DPS there is nothing wrong with your back. There is nothing wrong with your neck. There is nothing wrong with your shoulder, knees, legs, elbows, feet, or any other part of your body. The problem is rarely medical. The cause is psychological and the cure is to understand and accept the psychology of DPS. The faster you allow yourself to understand the real cause now, the faster you can become permanently pain-free, today.

Understand again, the purpose of DPS is to divert your attention from unbearable emotions to something more accept-able, like pain. Does this mean the pain is in your head? No. The pain is real, sometimes excruciating, but the real cause of your intense pain is psychological.

This is simply a process of your unconscious mind cre-ating a physical result--pain--because your unconscious mind believes that it's more dangerous to confront your buried emo-tions than to experience debilitating pain. What is your uncon-scious mind? Your unconscious mind is everything you are not conscious of right...................... NOW. Were you conscious of your feet touching the floor? Probably not. Were you conscious of your breathing? Probably not. Were you conscious of your cells regenerating? Your eyes blinking? Your heart beating? Probably not. However, all those things were taking place out of your awareness, unconsciously. One of the characteristics of your unconscious mind is that it is illogical. Your unconscious mind believes that you would rather be doubled over in pain then deal with emotions considered dangerous. As I indicated earlier, consciously, you would probably much rather deal with these emotions, such as anger, rage, fear, or a multitude of oth-ers, than suffer with your pain.

Unfortunately, that's not the normal pattern of your unconscious mind. The great news is that when you do change your focus from the physical pain to the psychological emotions, regardless of what the MRI or X-ray shows, your DPS pain will disappear. Thousands and thousands of people have permanently healed their pain by using a linguistic-only process to understand and accept the real cause of your discomfort. You can then change your strategy to focus on the emotions, rather than on the physical pain. Your old unconscious strategy of burying the negative emotions that are not congruent with your self-image is now replaced by a new strategy. By making this change, you are taking conscious control of your unconscious process. This change will ensure that you will permanently banish your pain.

When your unconscious mind is aware that you are aware of the emotion, your pain instantly disappears. Unfortunately, most people have been convinced that structural abnormalities, such as bulging discs, herniated discs, scoliosis, along with many other structural issues, cause pain. Many of my clients come to me waving their MRI results as a badge of honor. "I have a herniated disc and that's the cause of my pain." I carefully explain to them, "Yes you do have a bulging disc or a herniated disc, but that is not the cause of your pain."

Studies consistently demonstrate that two out of three people who have never had pain have herniated or bulging discs. Yet they never have pain. How then can disc abnormalities be the cause of pain? The truth is discs are almost never the cause. The cause is a psycho-physical process called DPS. Your pain is easy to heal. Thankfully, after one *Zero Pain Now* session, virtually everyone leaves free of any limiting pain. I don't

Hoag Hospital & Cleveland Clinic

MRIs On 98 People With No History Of Back Pain:

34%

HAD NORMAL DISCS

66%

HAD BULGING DISCS OR HERNIATED DISCS

Source: Maureen C. Jensen
New England Journal of Medicine, 1994

cure them. They heal themselves. They heal themselves just as you can heal yourself, with knowledge, with understanding, and with acceptance. This is the proof your problem begins in your brain. Since understanding is how you become pain-free, the cause must originate in your brain.

Misinformation and misdiagnosing most back pain started innocently. Many years ago, people went to the doctor complaining of back (or whatever) pain. They were given an X-ray, which showed some structural abnormality. Perhaps some common structural issue, which is regarded as an abnormality. These people were given a diagnosis by their doctors, based on X-ray results, which concluded that their pain was caused by their abnormality. In other words, their abnormal structure caused them to experience pain. Unfortunately, there was no basis for the diagnosis. It was simply guesswork that has led to one of the biggest epidemics in history. This epidemic is correctable and curable only with understanding.

The epidemic of back pain, neck pain, or more generally persistent pain anywhere in your body, will be changed when you understand and accept the real cause of your pain--DPS. In the words of Dr. John Sarno, the originator of the psychological diagnosis for physical pain, "Conventional medicine has failed." They have failed to make the complete diagnosis. This failure to diagnose correctly has created an estimated $600 billion per year industry in the United States alone. An article in Reuters stated the back-pain industry grew 65% in the last decade.

I recently searched on Google for back-pain products. The result was an astounding 17,600,000 possible sites. Every product was based on the false assumption that anatomy is causing pain. The advertised products included braces, shoes, inserts, special chairs, magnets, pillows, creams, herbs, vitamins, mattresses, cushions, exercise equipment, ice packs, heating devices, massagers, immobilizers, and many more items aimed at not curing your pain, but managing pain.

Prescription drugs have their own issues. When I see the name brand commercials promoting various prescription drugs, I am amazed, like you, at the long list of side effects. The misnomer is that pharmaceutical companies and the FDA would not allow a drug that would hurt the public out on the market. What about Vioxx? All drugs can be hazardous. According to a study completed by Gary Null, PhD adverse reactions to prescription drugs are responsible for more than 106,000 deaths every year. That's the size of the entire city where I grew up! Are prescribed drugs dangerous? Ask the families and friends of the people who've died.

The common pain diagnosis is based on a fallacy, and that fallacy is that structural issues are usually the cause of pain. This is unproven, and in my opinion, it is simply untrue. The truth is almost all persistent pain has a psychological cause and the name of the diagnosis is DPS. The purpose of DPS is to divert your attention from your buried emotions to something physical. In your case--physical pain.

Maureen Jensen published a study in the prestigious *New England Journal of Medicine* in 1994. MRIs were performed on ninety-eight people with no history of back pain. Thirty-four percent had what would be considered normal and healthy discs. Sixty-six percent had bulging discs at one or more levels, or disc protrusions or disc extrusions (herniated discs). How is this possible? If two out of three people who have never had pain have disc abnormalities, how can these structural issues be blamed for causing your pain? What does this mean? It means that disc problems almost never cause pain. It means most of what you have probably been told about the cause of your pain is false. Nearly two-thirds of the people in the study had the same structural abnormalities as you probably have, yet they've never had any pain. There are other studies that have similar results.

Scientific studies have been performed by top professionals and the results are incredibly similar. Two out of three people who have never experienced back pain, neck pain, shoulder pain, leg, knee or arm pain, have the same disc structural abnormalities but no pain. This is proof that the real cause of pain is not structural. The real cause of almost all persistent or chronic pain is psychological. The pain is real, physical, and can be excruciating. The diagnosis is usually DPS. The purpose of DPS is to divert your attention from psychological emotions to something physical. The sooner you decide to understand and believe the truth about the cause of your pain, the sooner you will experience the freedom when you decide to believe this, and rid yourself of the pain now.

Doctors at the University of Copenhagen compared X-rays of 238 patients with low back pain to sixty-six people with no history of back pain. They reported no structural difference. You are seeing a pattern, aren't you? Prestigious, scientific and professionally performed studies consistently show that there is no difference in the bodily structure of people with pain and people without pain. It becomes very simple for you to deduce that if your anatomy is the same as people without pain, anatomy or structure is not the cause of your pain. Again, here is more powerful proof that structure is not the culprit. Yes, the MRIs are accurate. People have disc bulges. Yes, people have herniated discs, stenosis and a host of other labeled "disc abnormalities." Yes, these studies continue to demonstrate to you that the real cause of your pain is not physical but psychological. And YES, you can heal your pain when you accept the psychology of DPS. As you begin to focus your attention on your emotions, you will begin to heal your pain.

Let's now discuss the topic of "placebo." A placebo is a treatment that is based on blind faith, meant to help or cure an ailment. Something similar to using a sugar pill instead of a drug. While I have witnessed that many people have extraordinary medical breakthroughs with placebo, pain is rarely a medical issue. Pain usually has a psychological cause. Treatments using placebos are rarely beneficial, and any positive results are usually temporary. In my opinion, most back surgeries are nothing more than a placebo. Thousands of unnecessary and unproductive surgeries are performed every year.

How many stories have you heard about people having back surgery, and after the surgery either the pain still exists, the pain is much worse (usually blamed on scar tissue), or some new pain has appeared elsewhere? Many of my clients have had surgery, (sometimes three or four surgeries) yet they still experience pain. In other clients, pain has appeared in new or different areas of their bodies. This is consistent with DPS theory. Surgeons are treating a symptom but not the cause. Therefore, any benefit is only the placebo effect and usually limited and temporary. The purpose of DPS is to divert your attention from emotional issues, such as anger or rage, to physical issues such as pain. Since the surgery only attacks the symptom, pain, your brain will find another diversion from your buried emotions. It's very common for someone to have had back surgery and later develop neck pain or pain in some other area. Performing surgery for most back, neck, shoulder, etc., pain can be compared to having a surgeon operate and remove the bulb when your oil warning light in your car is illuminated. A sort of "bulbectomy." By doing so you have performed surgery on the symptom. However, the cause still exists. It is only when you understand and accept the psychology of DPS that you will banish the pain forever.

A study was conducted by the Baylor School of Medicine in 1992, and published in the *New England Journal of Medicine*. The study involved people with major knee pain. The intent of the study was to determine which knee surgery is most effective and would provide the most relief. The study included three groups of patients. In the first group, Dr. Mosley shaved the damaged cartilage in the patient's knee. In the second group, the material thought to be causing the problem was flushed and removed. The third group received no surgery. These patients were given anesthesia, received standard incisions, and splashed water as if the full surgery, including flushing, were being performed. Forty minutes later, Mosley closed the incisions, pretending a complete surgery had been performed. The results were staggeringly surprising. All three groups showed the same improvement. Over 600,000 arthritic knee surgeries are performed annually. However, Dr. Mosley's study deems them to be unnecessary.

The epidemic of pain is not a medical problem, it's a psychological problem. This means just like the rest of us, you're human. We all repress emotions that aren't congruent with our self-image. In some people, like us, this results in pain. Your problem is caused by an old process of thinking and this is the reason you're still in pain. As you change the way you think, and begin to focus on your emotions, you allow yourself to be completely convinced that DPS is the cause of your pain. You now understand that it is a harmless condition whose purpose is to divert your attention from your emotional issues to physical pain. As you continue this new way of thinking, your pain will cease.

As I indicated earlier, we all experience psycho-physical reactions on a regular basis. In your case the result is pain. However, psycho-physical reactions can and do also lead to many gastrointestinal problems or disturbances. These are considered to be "equivalents" of DPS because they serve the same purpose as DPS. The purpose is to divert your attention from psychological emotions such as anger and rage to something physical. We all know our bodies and brains are one and connected. Science has proven there is a connection between your thoughts, your thought processes, and your body.

Experience has shown that approximately 88% of people with DPS pain also have a history of some form of gastrointestinal ailment. A few of the more common ailments are: reflux or heartburn, chronic constipation, irritable bowel syndrome, peptic ulcer, along with many others. The common denominator between these ailments and DPS pain is that the cause is thought to be emotional.

Hoag Hospital in Newport Beach, California and the Cleveland Clinic published a study in the *New England Journal of Medicine* in 1994. They reported finding lumbar disc bulges and protrusions on MRIs in sixty-four of ninety-eight people who never had back pain. Once again sixty-four of the ninety-eight people had never experienced any back pain. If the sixty-four people had major structural abnormalities, yet they never experienced any pain, you would have to be very silly to continue to believe that the cause of your pain is anything other than DPS.

You'll only heal your symptom when you fully accept that the cause of your pain is psychological. Don't believe the cause of your pain is psychological unless you want to heal yourself, now!

Who gets DPS? While anyone can have DPS, I have found most people fall into at least one of the following categories:

- Perfectionist
- Dependable
- Do-Gooders
- Spiritual-Religious
- People who need to be liked
- Seekers of new challenges
- Compulsive
- People Pleasers
- Control Freaks

I suspect you see some or many of these qualities in yourself. The reason is simple. Let's say you're a perfectionist, or if you're not willing to admit to being a perfectionist, let's just say you're very dependable. You like to do things the "right way." An obvious show of anger probably doesn't fit very well with the way you want to be seen. So when your spouse, your client, your parent or one of your kids says or does something that you don't like, instead of acknowledging the anger, you simply push it down and go forward. How about the good spiritual people out there. It's not okay to be angry--it's all about love and helping and being liked by others. Anger? No way! So the emotions are repressed. When those unbearable, "dangerous" emotions threaten to erupt into consciousness, bam! Your brain diverts your attention to physical pain. It's a scenario that plays over and over again.

Many of my clients have told me that they show anger. They yell at their spouse. They scream when someone cuts them off while driving. They show anger in many areas of their life. This is not the emotion that is causing your pain. This anger is conscious. The emotion that is causing your pain is unconscious. You are not yet aware of this emotion.

The pain stops when you refuse the diversion tactic and focus on your buried emotions. When you uncover the buried emotion, you will become pain-free.

Annie contacted me from Europe. Her story is very typical. Annie had been suffering pain for over twenty years. She had fallen off a horse more than twenty years earlier. She had been diagnosed with a broken tailbone that was now at a ninety degree inward angle. She was told it needed to be surgically corrected. Her pain had developed into a predictable pattern. She was able to sit for a very short time and then came pain. When she would stand, the pain would be extreme and decrease in intensity after a few minutes. As time went on the problem became more severe. In 1997 she was in a car accident. She was diagnosed with whiplash. According to the "experts," the whiplash syndrome was still causing pain thirteen years later. In 2005, she broke her shoulder. An orthopedic surgeon performed surgery, which was determined to be unsuccessful. The doctors performed another surgery. However, five years later, the pain persisted.

In 2008, Annie had another fall off a horse. She tore a ligament in her knee. Surgery was performed. Two years later, her knee was still swollen. She had developed a pattern that any time she did anything out of her ordinary routine, the pain became worse. Annie was desperate. Her life was limited. She asked me if I could help her finally get rid of the pain. She told me she had done everything. After she was diagnosed with DPS, I agreed to help her. I asked her if she was willing to accept the possibility that the cause of all her pain with psychological. I received a resounding yes.

We made an appointment for her session. Our session was conducted using Skype video conferencing software. Almost everyone's session follows a standard format. I began by teaching Annie all about DPS. I showed her all the facts, all the studies and the data that prove that the Path to Pain is a psycho-physical process. I told her that your DPS is simply your brain's way to divert your attention from unbearable emotions to physical pain. After approximately an hour, we began the final technique. I asked her on a level of one to ten what her current level of pain was? She responded with a "seven." She was propped up on pillows and she was in obvious pain. Over the course of thirty-five minutes, her pain went from seven, to a three, and then to a zero. Her pain was completely gone. Over twenty years of intense pain in many areas of her body, surgeries, drugs, alternative procedures, all the pain had been banished in thirty-five minutes. This is very common. When you finally understand the cause of your pain and then completely accept the psychology of DPS, your pain will disappear.

People often ask me, why does the pain come when it does? The answer is, The pain comes when the unbearable emotions threaten to burst into consciousness. Your brain picked that exact moment to divert your attention and deliver to you an old-fashioned dose of pain. This can occur when you are participating in a physical activity, moving something, or for no apparent reason. Sometimes the pain begins slowly and builds, or sometimes you experience an immediate burst of pain.

However, the cause is the same. When there is danger of your becoming conscious of the emotions, your brain will provide you with a diversion. Usually this diversion is physical pain.

Your brain is very smart. Since your unconscious mind has a blueprint for your entire body, it's not a surprise that your pain is often located at the place of a structural abnormality or a previous injury. Remember, the point of DPS is to divert your attention. It's a brain trick. So your brain is certainly going to do a good job of convincing your conscious mind by placing the pain at the point of a structural abnormality. Sometimes attacks of DPS arise slowly, while other times they come on suddenly, when you are doing something physical. Something such as lifting, or playing a sport. One time I was playing squash (a racket sport similar to racquetball) and at the very moment I took a big swing, I experienced extreme pain in my lower back. Most people would automatically suspect an injury. However, I knew better. I knew that DPS was the culprit. I knew this was my brain providing intense pain to keep me from focusing on some dangerous emotions. While it was extremely difficult, since my back was in excruciating pain, to focus on my emotions, I knew that was a requirement for getting better. I immediately left the court and quizzed myself on what emotions I was not paying attention to. Within moments I acknowledged the anger or perhaps better stated, the rage that I was feeling. The pain disappeared as quickly as it arose. I've seen so many other people suffer through long-term pain, even surgery, after similar episodes.

Now that you are familiar with DPS, you understand its purpose, you understand the Path to Pain and why you are in pain, what do you do to get out of the pain? Your healing your pain involves four components: understand the real cause of your pain, accept that DPS is the cause of your pain, follow the process to become pain-free, and continue to think psychologically in the future to stay free of pain.

You now understand DPS. Hopefully, you do believe that DPS is the cause of your pain. Now I will explain the steps to becoming pain-free. I titled this "The Highway To Healing."

The Highway to Healing is your direct route to finally ending this old pattern of pain and moving forward to freedom.

The first step in the Highway to Healing is to renounce the anatomical or structural diagnosis. You now have the knowledge to absolutely renounce this misdiagnosis. The facts and studies I have provided you, have allowed you to be convinced that the real cause of your pain is not structural.

The second step on your Highway to Healing is to acknowledge that the real cause of your pain is psychological emotions. You are very familiar with the process and it is easy for you to acknowledge that repressed emotions lead to your old pain.

This leads you to the third step on your Highway to Healing, the step that will really begin to propel you to feeling better. The third step is for you to focus on your emotions. As you focus on the emotions, you will bring to light the buried emotions, such as anger and rage, that have been in the dark and out of your awareness. You shine a bright light in the darkness of your unconscious mind by focusing that light (your attention) on your buried emotions.

The next step is to speak out loud to your brain. Yes, I know, if done in the wrong public environment, people will think that you are crazy. This can lead you to exit the Highway to Healing and take you straight to a mental institution. However, this is a very important and extremely powerful step in becoming pain-free. Many of my clients have used this and had astonishing results. I was explaining this step to my friend Debbie. She was an occasional sufferer of TMJ (temporomandibular joint disorder) pain. The next time she experienced pain, she said to her brain, "I know what you are doing. I know you are trying to divert my attention from my emotions to pain.

I get it. It's not going to work, so stop it now!" Her pain disappeared on the spot. Speak out loud to your brain. It works.

The final step on your Highway to Healing is one that only you can decide when to take. Almost all of my clients come to me as a referral from doctors. They have been properly diagnosed with DPS. Therefore, there is nothing wrong with their back, neck, shoulder, knee, foot, or any other part of their body. There is absolutely no danger in their commencing regular physical activity. Therefore, it is imperative for you to become and stay pain-free, you must resume regular physical activity. Since you probably have not been sent to me by a doctor, you may have used the information in this book to diagnose yourself. It is your responsibility to decide what and how much physical activity is best for you. The sooner you are able to commence regular physical activity, the sooner you will banish DPS pain.

The Highway to Healing will lead you to what is, in my opinion, the most wonderful destination in the world: freedom, a resumption of a full life, and lots of smiles. It's a trip worth taking, now.

You have learned and processed a great deal of information in this chapter. You comprehend the Path to Pain. You recognize how the Path led you to pain. You are now an expert in the simple process of DPS. If I asked you to tell me about why you are in pain, you would begin by telling me that you have DPS. You would continue to state that DPS is a psycho-physical process. It begins as psychological and leads to physical changes.

The Path to Pain starts by repressing or burying emotions that your unconscious mind considered to be too dangerous or unbearable. You'd continue to tell me that this produces a change in your autonomic nervous system. Your blood vessels became a little smaller. This reduces the amount of blood flowing through the vessels. Since oxygen is carried in blood, with less blood, there is less oxygen. Therefore, you would tell me that the real cause of pain is a slight oxygen deprivation. You would continue to tell me that the purpose of DPS is to divert your attention from your psychological emotions to physical symptoms, usually pain.

Since you know that you are an expert, you would continue and now tell me how to become pain-free. You would undoubtedly begin with the Highway to Healing. The first step is to renounce the anatomical or structural diagnosis. Then acknowledge that the real cause is psychological emotions. You'd continue to tell me to focus on my emotions and speak out loud to my brain. Then as soon as practicable, to recommence regular physical activity. This will lead to freedom, a resumption of a full life, and lots more smiles.

WOW! You really know this stuff. You followed the instructions and read every word of this book in order, and understand and accept the psychology of DPS.

HIGHWAY TO HEALING

RENOUNCE ANATOMICAL *OR STRUCTURAL* DIAGNOSIS

ACKNOWLEDGE REAL CAUSE *IS* PSYCHOLOGICAL

FOCUS ON YOUR EMOTIONS

SPEAK WITH YOUR BRAIN

COMMENCE REGULAR ACTIVITY

FREEDOM • BACK TO LIFE • MORE SMILES

Congratulations! Now it is time for you to

BANISH YOUR PAIN.

"In 10 minutes, 80% of my pain was gone."

Adam and his wife came over for dinner at my house one night. After cooking all day, my back spasms were so bad I was bent over in pain. I'd been in consistent pain for two months, and had occasional severe pain for thirty years. I always believed that I had a bad back.

As I sat down next to Adam complaining about the pain, he commented, "You have the perfect personality for back pain." When I asked him to explain, he described the basics of Diversion Pain Syndrome, and within about 10 minutes, 80% of my pain was gone. I scheduled a session with Adam, and within 30 days I had no more back pain. His treatment completely changed my life. There were so many activities I missed out on because of my chronic back pain. Now, I do ballet, run, hike and have no limitations! He literally transformed my life.

— **ANNEE DELLA DONNA**
Attorney
Laguna Beach, CA

NOTES

7

BANISH YOUR PAIN NOW

If you can read one more chapter, digest a few more pages, give all your attention to, and do one more exercise, and finally become free of your pain, will that be worthwhile to you? If you can give all your focus and dedication to go through a simple process that has helped hundreds of people cure their pain, some in as little as twenty minutes, are you willing?

There is a scene in the movie "Rambo." The camera shows Rambo looking out about four or five football fields away. He sees tanks, multiple helicopters with missiles ready, hundreds of men with just about every type of armor, all ready to use against him. Rambo looks exhausted. The tension is everywhere. His friend asks him, "What are you gonna do?" Rambo takes a long look at the enemy force, cocks his gun, and sternly says, "F' em!" He then takes off directly towards the enemies, running and shooting. This is the approach you must bring to this process. The more pain you have and the longer you have suffered, the more difficult it is to focus on your buried emotions. You must look at the enemy and say "F' em!"

You have done an amazing job so far. You have demonstrated your dedication and determination by reading every word of every page in this book. You have learned new things. You have transformed your limiting beliefs about your pain into new powerful beliefs. You have shifted your old strategy of repressing emotions into a new strategy, where you consciously focus on your emotions. You acknowledge all of your emotions. You are not the same person you were when you began reading this book. You have created a new world for yourself. Perhaps the level of your pain has changed. Regardless of how much pain exists now, you are ready to say good-bye to your old limiting pain, and say hello to your new, amazing life.

Everything you have read, everything you have learned, all your new thinking, has prepared you for this. If you do not do this exercise and just complete the mandatory homework in the next chapter, you will probably still be able to heal your pain sometime in the next month. Thousands of people have healed their DPS pain in just that way.

I had a client who came to me after thirty-six years of

pain. Let's call her Mary. Mary had surgery at age twelve. The surgery failed. She had been suffering since. The pain began in her back. As time went along, the pain spread to other areas of her body. She came to my office for a session. As always, I spent about an hour teaching her about the real cause of her pain. I provided her the same information that you have already learned while reading this book. As I have already indicated to you many times, the way you heal your DPS pain is with knowledge. You understand that the purpose of DPS is to divert your attention from your psychological emotions to physical symptoms, such as pain. When you understand and accept that the pain is caused by a slight oxygen deprivation, you are ready to begin to focus on the emotions and heal your pain.

After I explained DPS to Mary, and she understood completely, we began the process you are about to learn. Mary used the process to uncover the buried emotion(s) that were causing her pain for the last thirty-six years. The entire process took less than thirty-five minutes. Suddenly, she displayed the smile that makes my career so worthwhile. The smile that says, I am pain-free. I feel great. You said this would happen and it really did happen. The pain just went away. Mary's entire world changed, because something that used to be unbelievable is now her truth. She healed herself. I didn't heal her. I'm your teacher and tour guide. You heal yourself.

Within three hours of leaving my office, Mary was at the gym, exercising! The following are a portion of her words taken from an e-mail she sent me the next day;

Adam, Yes, I enjoyed working with you yesterday as well. And ~ Yes I was so inspired and went to the gym and did a Pilates Mat class (1 HR) and then ran on the elliptical for 30 minutes. A good start. Today I am going over to take either a Water Range of Motion class or a Gentle Yoga class. I think what you are doing is Wonderful! I look forward to this journey of becoming more conscious emotionally.

Keep shining your light!--Mary

The healing Mary gave herself is common. Most of my clients share similar stories. Everything Mary did for herself, you can do for yourself, today, right now. This process works. Make it work for you.

As you now completely understand, your pain is a result of a flawed strategy that you have used in the past to repress or bury what your unconscious mind considered to be "unbearable" emotions. You have had months, years, or perhaps even decades of practicing your old strategy. It will take your best "Rambo" determination to allow yourself to uncover the buried emotions that have caused your pain. It is safe for you to become aware of your repressed emotions. It is safe for you to become aware of your repressed emotions. IT IS SAFE, for you to become aware of your repressed emotions. They are just emotions. As you allow yourself to consciously feel what you are feeling, you will remove your pain. Some of my clients try to make it hard work. It isn't. Allow yourself to make it easy. It is.

One of my favorite clients lives in Europe. He is a big, strong, ex-rugby player. A real tough-looking guy. He prided himself on always being positive. No unconscious negative emotions for this guy. Except, he could barely get out of bed because of his back pain. When he was ready for the process you are about to learn, he contacted me and we began. He was determined not to become aware of the emotion(s). He kept telling me all he felt was pain. He would say, "No emotion, just blank." We must have gone back and forth for over an hour before he chose to let the emotions become conscious - before he allowed himself to become aware of the emotions. Once he let go, the negative emotions flowed freely. Finally, I asked him to tell me his level of discomfort. He stood up. He bent over. He stretched. He contorted his body. Then, he flashed me the smile and said one word, "Gone." His results were great. He healed his pain. However, he worked way harder that necessary. If you allow the emotions to flow, and permit yourself to become easily aware of them, you will make this process and your life much easier.

Let this part of the *Zero Pain Now* Process work for you. As I earlier indicated, with the information you already understand about DPS, you can perform the mandatory tasks in the next chapter to rid yourself of pain. However, if you are like me, you want to make the pain go away fast. How about right now?

This part of the process is very simple. The entire exercise consists of one question. That's it. One question. In my experience with helping so many people heal their pain, this question will allow you to "force the issue." By answering this one question in a very specific way, you will be able to uncover and make yourself consciously aware of, the emotion(s) that have been causing your pain. You already know that the purpose of DPS is to divert your attention from psychological emotions to physical symptoms. So what will happen when you use this question and allow yourself to become aware of your emotion(s)? There will be no emotion(s) from which to divert your attention. If there is no need to divert, there is no pain. When you use this question to quickly access your buried emotion(s) you will be pain-free.

Are you ready? Here is the question;

Right now, what emotion are you feeling?

I know, I know. You read this entire book. You learned everything you need to know about the real cause of your pain. You one-hundred-percent believe and accept that the cause of your pain is DPS, and this is the grand finale?

Yes. This is the question you will use in a very specific way to uncover the buried emotions that have caused your pain. Every client who has ever come to me has used this question to quicken their Highway to Healing. You will use this question as a shortcut to uncovering your emotions and to healing your pain.

Here is what you do. It must be done exactly as I describe for you to get the maximum benefit.

You can do this part of the process by yourself or you can ask someone to help you. I believe it is much easier to work with someone else. When you work with someone else, you are free to completely focus on exposing the emotions. Will it work for you alone? As long as you let it work for you, it will work for you. If you can find someone to help you, do it. For those of you who believe that you hate to ask others for help, this is the time to step through your limiting beliefs and ask for assistance. While the exercise can work with a spouse or significant other, I recommend using someone else. If the source of the buried emotion has something to do with him or her, you may limit yourself. Whoever you decide, get some help. How important is healing your pain?

I will first describe the process as a two-person process. This is the way I help clients in my office. I will then describe the process for one person. Please thoroughly and completely read both methods. The two-person method is preferred.

The Two-Person Method

Have both participants sit comfortably. You can sit on a chair or a couch. It does not matter as long as you are comfortable. You can face one another or sit next to each other. Just as long as you are comfortable. The person you have chosen to help you needs a pad of paper, or something to write down your answers. Before you begin, have your partner ask you, on a scale of one to ten, with one being very little pain and ten being excruciating pain, what is your current level of discomfort? Have them write down your answer.

The exercise begins with your partner in a neutral voice, asking you, "Right now, what emotion are you feeling? "

You answer, "I am feeling _____. "
You must answer with a real emotion.

I've had so many people answer, "I'm feeling pain."
I answer, "Good, but pain is not an emotion."

I then repeat the question.

"Right now, what emotion are you feeling?"

When you answer the question, your partner will write the name of the emotion on the piece of paper.

Then your partner will repeat the question.

"Right now, what emotion are you feeling?"

You will answer,"I am feeling _____."

You may answer with the same emotion, or you may be feeling a different emotion. Just answer with whatever emotion you are feeling at that moment.

You must always begin your answer with, I am feeling. Have your partner pay attention so if you leave out the I am feeling, they can remind you.

This continues exactly the same way.

They ask, "Right now, what emotion are you feeling?" You reply with, "I am feeling _____" filling in the blank with the emotion you are feeling.

Your partner will then say one of two things, "Good," then repeat the question.

Or, "Good, _____ is not an emotion."

Then repeat the question.

After asking the question twenty or twenty-five times, your partner will ask, "What is your current level of discomfort?"

Sometimes the pain goes down in a linear fashion towards

zero. Other times the level of pain goes up and down as you get close to uncovering the emotion(s). This is because sometimes your brain raises the level of pain as a final effort to keep the emotion out of your awareness.

Any change in your level of pain is more proof that the cause of your pain is psychological.

Questions and answers do not change your spine. Whether linear or up and down, either way is perfect. The number is just a gauge to know where you are in the process.

Many of my clients have found the process to be much easier when they close their eyes and focus their attention on the area of their body from their stomach to their chest. This is the area most people feel negative emotions. Focusing here will probably help you expedite the exercise. This is not a conscious process. It is not about thinking. Therefore, focusing your attention around your chest and stomach area will also help you "stay out of your head."

Since DPS is really a strategy of disconnecting from your emotions, many "thinkers" initially have difficulty connecting with emotions. Allow yourself to feel what's there. I had one client diagnosed with a torn rotator cuff. He had been suffering with this incarnation of DPS for two months. Many sleepless nights and painful days preceded his session with me. Every time he was considering a career change, he would experience symptoms. He had already had neck surgery and many other pain and gastrointestinal problems. He just could not feel negative emotions. Since I knew he had a sister, I knew he must have been angry in the past! I had him remember a specific time when he was furious at his sister. After a few minutes his physiology changed and he felt the rage. I asked him to pay attention to the feeling. Now I asked him to think of something currently that has him angry. As he thought of the current situation he was able to connect the feeling from the past to the current event. He could now recognize how the feelings of anger and rage felt in his body. Within ten minutes, his shoulder pain dropped from an eight to a one.

Another tip is to continue to focus on the negative emotions. Many of my clients have spent decades perfecting the art of feeling positive emotions. It is very unlikely that the emotions causing your pain are happiness or joy. Focus on the anger, rage, and the other negative emotions. Take whatever emotions surface. It may not make sense. That's perfectly okay. Whatever you get is perfect, as long as they are negative emotions. Just feel what you feel.

This is the entire exercise. Please perform the exercise exactly as I have described. When do you stop? When the pain is gone. How much time will you need? As long as it takes. With my clients, I've spent as little as fifteen minutes, and as long as three hours, until the pain was gone.

Years ago I was using this process as an experiment with my wife. For the record, I've learned that experiment and wife are not the best combination. She had a tension headache. So of course I'm coming to the rescue with my *Zero Pain Now* Process. She already knew the basics, so we jumped right in to this part of the process.

I began asking her, "Right now, what emotion are you feeling?" She answered, "I am feeling _____."

"What emotion are you feeling right now?"
"I am feeling _____."

"Right now, what emotion are you feeling?"
"I am feeling _____."
Her level of pain was rising.

After about ten minutes, I looked at my watch and said, "Sorry Honey, I need to get to the office...We'll finish up later." What started as a manageable tension headache was now a roaring firebomb of a headache, and I just left her. When do you stop? When the pain is gone. Give yourself enough time. No interruptions. No kids. No dogs. Stop only when the pain is gone.

The One-Person Method

Begin by sitting comfortably either on a couch or on a chair. It doesn't matter as long as you are comfortable. You need a pad of paper to write down your answers. Before you begin the exercise, ask yourself, On a level of one to ten, with one being very little pain and ten being excruciating pain, what is my current level of discomfort? Write the number on the paper.

Begin the exercise by asking yourself out loud, "Right now, what emotion am I feeling?"

Then answer, "I am feeling _____."

You must answer with a real emotion.

I've had so many people answer, "I'm feeling pain." I answer, "Good, but pain is not an emotion."

I then repeat the question.

Jot the name of the emotion on the paper.

Then repeat the question.

"Right now, what emotion am I feeling?"

You will answer, "I am feeling _____."

You must begin your answer with, I am feeling.

Pay attention so if you leave out the I am feeling, you will catch yourself.

This continues exactly the same way.

Ask yourself out loud, "Right now, what emotion am I feeling?"

You reply with, "I am feeling _____", filling in the blank with the emotion you are feeling.

You will then say, out loud, one of two things; "Good," then repeat the question.

Or, "Good, _____ is not an emotion."

Then repeat the question.

After asking the question twenty or twenty-five times, ask yourself, "What is my current level of discomfort?" Sometimes the pain goes down in a linear fashion towards zero. Other times the level of pain goes up and down as you get close to uncovering the emotion(s). This is because sometimes your brain raises the level of pain as a final effort to keep the emotion out of your awareness.

Any change in your level of pain is more proof that the

cause of your pain is psychological. Questions and answers do not change your spine. Whether linear or up and down, either way is perfect. The number is just a gauge to know where you are in the process.

Many of my clients have found the process to be much easier when they close their eyes and focus their attention on the area of their bodies from their stomachs to their chests. This is the area most people feel negative emotions. Focusing here will probably help you expedite the exercise. This is not a conscious process. It is not about thinking. Therefore, focusing your attention around your chest and stomach area will also help you "stay out of your head." Another tip is to continue to focus on the negative emotions. Many of my clients have spent decades perfecting the art of feeling positive emotions. It is very unlikely that the emotions causing your pain are happiness or joy. Focus on the anger, rage, and the other negative emotions. Take whatever emotions surface. It may not make sense. That's perfectly OK. Whatever you get is perfect as long as they are negative emotions. Just feel what you feel.

This is the entire exercise. Please perform the exercise exactly as I have described. When do you stop? When the pain is gone. How much time will you need? As long as it takes. With my clients, I've spent as little as fifteen minutes, and as long as three hours, until the pain was gone. Stop only when the pain is gone.

As I indicated, it is important to know what is an emotion and what is not an emotion. Interestingly, I've found the buried emotions that are causing the pain are almost always anger, or more specifically, rage.

Here is a partial list of negative emotions:
- Anger
- Rage
- Hurt
- Sadness
- Fear
- Guilt
- Shame
- Jealous
- Disgust
- Anxiety
- Resentment
- Disappointment
- Envy
- Frustration
- Worry
- Exasperated
- Disgust
- Irritated
- Panic
- Envy
- Overwhelm
- Harassed
- Embarrassed
- Annoyed

I don't recall anyone ever becoming pain-free experiencing an emotion that is not on this list. As I said, the emotions usually responsible are anger and/or rage. Many people initially notice emotions that seem less threatening, such as frustration, or annoyed. Eventually, as you continue to dig, you will uncover the deeper, more "unbearable" emotions such as anger and rage.

Here are some examples of what are not emotions:

- Pain is not an emotion
- Loser is not an emotion
- Failure is not an emotion
- Stupid is not an emotion
- Alone is not an emotion
- Undeserving is not an emotion
- Unlovable is not an emotion
- Pain is not an emotion (Yes, I used this twice, because it's such a common mistake.)

If you are following my recommendation, and have chosen to work with a partner, good choice. Even if you are going to do the process by yourself, I'd like you to take some time before you begin and do a couple of tasks. Consider this "Metamucil" for your emotions. Take out some paper and make a list of everything that adds or has added stress in your life. Yes, this is a very long list. This is not the time to be spiritual or censor yourself in any way. Add everything you can recall. When you have completed, add more. I promise you it's there.

When you are really complete, and everything is on

the list, spend AT LEAST FIFTEEN MINUTES writing about whatever is on the list. Spelling and punctuation don't matter. Just free write about anything and everything that provide you with stress, tension, anger, rage, etc. Let it flow as fast as you can. You may notice as you do this that your level of pain changes.

The exercise has been a complete success for about 85% of my clients. The rest just took a bit longer. A few of you will have reduced your level of pain, and will need to perform the tasks described in the next chapter to finish becoming pain-free. Yes, I understand this is in opposition to all my earlier statements and directives to keep going until the pain is gone. For most of you that is exactly how the exercise will play out. I described the process the way I did because I would much rather you go way, way, way, way too long than too short. The danger is in not going long enough and not becoming completely pain-free. The danger is in stopping too soon, and in not allowing yourself to assure your success and completely banish your pain. Your chances are great that you will banish your pain as long as you do not stop the exercise until your pain is gone. When you have completed the list and only when you have completed it, do the exercise. Stop reading now, make your list and do the exercise.

Continue the exercise until you banish your pain. Flash your partner, or yourself, the famous "I feel great" smile, and then read on.

8

WHAT SHOULD I DO NOW?

In the previous chapter I told you a little about Mary. She was in pain for thirty-six years. In one short session, Mary was able to completely heal her pain and become pain-free. As you already read, she was at the gym, exercising and had returned to all normal physical activities.

I always ask my clients to send me daily updates, so I know they are remaining free of pain, and to confirm that they are doing the mandatory follow-up tasks. Mary was not sending me her daily notes. After a few weeks, I reached out to her through e-mail to inquire as to how she was doing. Here was her reply: I am doing all the stuff but am in pain..... well, not doing the 15 min of saying out loud how I am feeling.

"No Surgery for me."

I was told that I needed disc surgery. I was terrified and willing to do anything to avoid surgery. I heard about Adam and his *Zero Pain Now* Process. I called Adam and arranged a referral from my M.D. to meet with him. I was more than a little leery because his promise sounded too good to be true. He told me if I didn't cure my own pain, my session was free. After one hour of Adam teaching me about the cause of my pain, he began asking me some very basic questions. For the first time in years, my pain disappeared. He gave me some tasks to do at home, and I'm still pain-free.

— **TONY SANDERS**
Investor
New York, NY

I was flabbergasted. Mary went through one short session and quickly put thirty-six years of debilitating and limiting pain in her past. She was given very specific instructions as to exactly what was necessary to transform her old repression strategy into a new strategy that would focus on emotions and keep her pain-free. She knew the process works because she had already experienced the success. She was free of pain! All she needed to do was complete the tasks and make the change permanent. Why didn't she?

Everyone motivates themselves in different ways. Some people are motivated by moving toward something. If your boss offers you an additional twenty percent bonus to increase your productivity, or to increase your sales, or to increase anything, would you be motivated toward receiving the bonus? If your answer is yes, your motivation is "Toward." You prefer to move towards a goal. You are motivated more by a carrot than a stick.

On the other hand, would you be more motivated if the boss said, "If you don't increase your productivity, you will be fired?" This is an example of an "Away from" motivation. A common example of "Away from" motivation is seen in many people attempting to lose weight. You undoubtedly know people who made the decision to lose weight. They started quickly and began losing weight. At some point they stopped losing weight, and they began gaining back the weight. This pattern is usually the result of an "Away from" motivation. They initially start losing weight because they don't want something. They don't want a heart attack. They don't want surgery. They don't want a stroke. They don't want to buy bigger clothes. Something they are motivated to move away from. What happens after they lose some weight? They emotionally move farther away from what they don't want. The fear that drove them away is not as strong, because they are not as close. Therefore, their motivation lessens. They lost some weight and feel further from the heart attack or the larger-size clothes. Since they are further from the situation that they are moving away from, there is less need, or less motivation, to continue.

You've seen this happen with friends, family or perhaps even yourself many times. So what about Mary? She came to me, desperate. She was in pain and was willing to do anything to "Move away" from the pain. She was motivated. She was determined. She went through the process and she was successful. What happened when Mary had no more pain? She was no longer motivated. She didn't do the mandatory tasks. She went back to her old pattern of thinking, and she brought back her pain.

Mary knows the process works because it already had.

Let's compare Mary's results with those of Rand. Rand was one of the approximately fifteen percent of people who were not completely free of pain at the end of doing the last exercise. His level of pain dropped considerably. Yet he still was experiencing pain. Instead of being disappointed, Rand was even more determined make his process work for himself.

He did every task I gave him. He was diligent. He not only did what I asked him to do, he asked for more. He sent me notes not just every day, but several times each day detailing his steady progress. Each day was a little better. On the sixth day after his session, he sent me a note comparing his absence of pain to when the flu breaks. He was driving home from the gym (he chose to resume normal physical activity immediately) and he realized there was no pain. It was completely gone. Rand knew there was nothing wrong with his back. He was determined to succeed, and he did. If you need to reinvigorate yourself, take a moment and reread Rand's success story at the beginning of the book.

If your pain is completely gone, do these follow-up tasks exactly as written. If your pain is not completely gone, it's okay. Just like Rand, you can use these tasks to complete the process and become pain-free. Thousands of people have healed their DPS pain without using the last exercise. If you stay "Rambo tough," you will heal your pain. So if your pain is gone, do the mandatory tasks to keep the pain away. If it isn't gone, do the mandatory tasks to make any remaining pain go away. There is one common denominator: Please do the mandatory tasks. Do them every day. Do them as long as required.

NOTES

Mandatory Tasks To Help You Become or Stay Free Of Pain

1. Schedule enough time every day to perform these tasks. Most of you have busy lives. You have plenty of daily activities and situations with which to keep busy. It's easy to fall behind. These tasks are extremely important. That's why I call them "mandatory tasks." Place every task every day in your Blackberry, iPhone, PDA, or any type of calendar. You will be much more likely to have success.

2. Any time you feel any pain, ask yourself and answer the question, out loud, until the pain is gone. As NLP Trainer Tad James said, "Let your pain be your guide." You probably had great success when you used this question in the earlier exercise. If you did not completely rid yourself of pain, you probably lessened your pain. This exercise works as long as you let it work. It's easier for some people to tune into their emotions. This is the easiest way I have found for you to uncover unconscious emotions. You are in the process of training your unconscious mind to perform a new strategy. Any time you feel any pain, immediately stop what you are doing and begin the question: Right now, what emotion am I feeling? Answer out loud, "I am feeling _____." Be sure your answer is a negative emotion, such as anger or rage. Remember to focus on the area near your stomach and chest. Continue asking and answering the question until the pain is gone.

3. For the next thirty days or until you have been pain-free for at least two weeks, whichever is LONGER, spend at least fifteen minutes at one time, every day, asking and answering the question. You are training your unconscious mind to perform a new strategy. Your new strategy is to focus on your emotions. This is the best way I have found to retrain your brain to think differently. If your pain is already gone, this takes discipline. This really works. Do this every day.

4. For the next thirty days, make a daily list of everything in your life that adds stress or tension. Make a new list every day. You will be amazed what you will continue to discover as you do this task every day. New things will arise. Some will be things you have not remembered in years... others will be things you hadn't yet considered. Take enough time to place everything on the list. When you think you are done, look again, look deeper. There is always more.

5. For the next thirty days, spend at least ten minutes each day writing about anything that adds stress to your life. This is different than making your list. Now you are free writing. Write about anything and everything that adds stress or tension. Write quickly. Grammar and spelling are unimportant. Don't censor yourself. Anything and everything you write is okay. You will see that when you do this task, other emotions and circumstances will emerge, and they will differ from your list. Perform this after you have done task number 4.

6. Speak out loud with your brain. This really works. Tell your brain you know what it is doing. Tell it that you know it is trying to divert your attention from your psychological emotions to physical symptoms. Tell your brain you are "on to" its process, and the game is over. Whatever words you use to speak to your brain are fine, as long as you speak out loud to your brain.

7. Think psychological. As you go through your days, remember to focus on your emotions. You may have learned over the last years or decades to repress or bury your emotions. You can also relearn to be aware of your emotions. Remind yourself to notice what you are feeling. You don't have to act on the emotions. You don't have to change the emotions. You do need to notice and acknowledge your emotions.

As you continue to perform these tasks, and I know you will perform them every day with zest and dedication, your life will change. You will have accomplished something. You will have changed your thinking. You will have shifted your world. You will be free of DPS pain. You will be free. And you will be smiling.

May you be blessed with a lifetime of smiles.

NOTES

9

ANSWERING YOUR QUESTIONS

As you go through your *Zero Pain Now* Process, questions will inevitably arise. I have listed some of the most commonly asked ones below.

In addition, many of my clients have asked for a companion workbook, audio, or video to help them quicken their healing. As I've emphasized throughout this book, daily action is critical to your success. Whatever helps you stay committed to those actions to digging deep and removing the underlying cause to your pain is a plus. You can see a sample of the video on our website which will demonstrate the techniques so you

are able to perform them precisely as I do in my one-on-one
sessions. The workbook provides additional helpful tasks, with
space for you to write the answers to the questions.

How Long Will It Take For Me To Be Free Of Pain?

In my experience most of my clients will either greatly
reduce their pain or become free of pain while answering the
question I gave you. Some people take longer. The benchmark
for improvement is different for everyone. It is not uncommon to experience some fluctuations in pain while you are
doing your follow-up tasks. Many people will stay permanently
pain-free after using the process. Others will still experience
pain (usually much less) for some period of time. It is not
uncommon to take three steps forward and then one step back.
Your unconscious mind will attempt to test you and keep you
in pain. Be vigilant. The longest I have seen a client take to
become pain-free was a man who came to me after having
seven unsuccessful surgeries, six on his spine. His level of pain
increased, decreased, and fluctuated for six weeks. His determination to stay with the process eventually led him to becoming
pain-free. Be persistent. Be determined. Stay with the tasks and
the process until you banish your pain.

How Can I Increase My Chances And Get Better Faster?

Remember that of most importance are your ability and willingness to believe that you have made the correct
diagnosis that your pain and discomfort has been caused by
Diversion Pain Syndrome. This belief will allow you to expe-

dite your healing. Everyone leaves my office certain that DPS is the cause of their pain. Sometimes they lose confidence in the diagnosis. They begin to consider the possibility that their bulging disc, or crooked back is the cause. They listen to their friends try to convince them that their problem is structural. If you choose to sit on the fence and look at both possibilities, your unconscious mind will continue to send you pain and the other symptoms of Diversion Pain Syndrome. Clients, including those who are most successful in responding to the *Zero Pain Now* Process, sometimes go through periods of doubt. The doubt is your unconscious mind's attempt to return to the process of diverting your attention away from what it perceives to be dangerous, or unbearable emotions. Learning to banish your doubt is part of the permanent cure. The more certain you are of your diagnosis, the faster you will permanently heal your symptoms and regain your freedom.

Will I Be Able To Resume Normal Physical Activities?

Once you have decided that Diversion Pain Syndrome is the real cause of your pain, you are well on your way to resuming a physical life without limitations. Since by definition DPS is a psycho-physical disorder that originates in your brain, it means there is nothing wrong with your back, your neck, your knee, elbow, foot, etc. Therefore resuming physical activities is not only possible, it will expedite your healing. Many of my clients participate in vigorous physical exercise within days of healing themselves in their *Zero Pain Now* Process session. My advice to you is to take it easy at first. Slowly prove to yourself that you are structurally fine, and that you are physically able to perform physical activities. Then enjoy your freedom.

Do I Need To Quit My Stressful Job or Change My Career?

The cause of your pain and other symptoms is never the stressful job, or traumatic relationship, or frustrating children. The cause is the way you dealt with the anger and other emotions. The cause of Diversion Pain Syndrome is the unconscious act of repressing emotions such as anger or rage. All that is required to banish your pain is to liberate the emotion. Since the purpose of DPS is to divert your attention from some dangerous or unbearable emotion to something physical, such as pain, when you consciously experience the emotion, your pain disappears. There is nothing left to divert.

This doesn't mean that you won't want to make some changes in your life to create as much happiness as you can. However, to free yourself from your pain, these life style changes are not necessary. Focus on your emotions and you will become and stay pain-free.

What Emotions Are Responsible For My Pain?

Any repressed emotion can be responsible for causing your Diversion Pain Syndrome symptoms. Fear, jealousy, guilt, shame, sadness and any other negative emotion can be the root cause of your problem. However, well over ninety percent of my clients have ended their battle with pain after discovering their buried anger and/or rage.

Anger and rage have been deemed inappropriate by society. Therefore, many of us are taught as children that anger and rage are bad. In addition, many religions and spiritual groups preach that negative emotions such as anger are wrong.

As sentient human beings, we are subject to a full range of emotions. Anybody with a spouse or partner, a job, children, parents, etc., has plenty of occasions every day to experience anger and even rage. I'm not suggesting that you express your feelings at your will. What I am asserting is that as long as you acknowledge your emotions, whatever they are, you will become, and stay, pain-free. Remember, the sole purpose of Diversion Pain Syndrome is to divert your attention from unbearable, dangerous emotions to something physical, such as pain. What you don't know WILL hurt you. Acknowledging your negative emotions is all you must do to become and stay free of pain.

How Does Fear Affect DPS?

While fear can be the emotion that causes your symptoms, as I have stated, most of the time repressed anger and/or rage are responsible.

Fear can play a major role both in exacerbating symptoms and delaying rapid healing. Before learning about this method to heal pain, many people believed that they had a "bad back." Therefore this limiting and false beliefs can lead to fear of exercise and other physical activities. Part of my definition of a complete cure is the absence of fear and the resumption of normal physical activities. Since understanding and believing that Diversion Pain Syndrome is the cause of your pain is paramount to your healing yourself, any residual fear of hurting yourself helps to keep you stuck in pain. When you understand and believe that there is nothing wrong with your back, neck, etc., you will have no fear of physical activity. The more you participate in physical activities, the faster you banish your fear.

Will Stomach and Core Exercises Help Me?

Stomach and core exercised are great for looking your best and general overall health. They do nothing to help you get out of DPS pain. In fact, if you are exercising as a method of managing your pain, the exercise regime will, in actuality, keep you stuck in pain.

Believing that your pain has a psychological cause is critical for you to rapidly heal your pain. If you are working on stomach and core muscles as a healing method, you are not yet convinced that DPS is the culprit. Nothing less than one-hun-dred-percent belief will enable you to permanently heal your pain.

I suggest that you temporarily discontinue any method

you have been using to treat your symptoms until you have been free from pain for at least two weeks. This includes exercise, massage, physical therapy, chiropractic adjustments and any other modalities. Always consult your physician before making any changes to your medical regime.

Stay with the exercises I've provided in this book. The more dedicated you are, the faster you will experience the freedom that comes with ending your pain and getting your full life back.

How Long Do I Need To Continue The Program After I Cure Myself?

Many people complete this program and never feel another symptom. When you change your thinking and your pain disappears, what would happen if you went back to your old way of thinking and processing emotions? You could bring back symptoms. Once in a while I feel some pain in my lower back. I take this as a reminder to pay attention and focus on my emotions. I immediately ask myself, "Right now, what emotion am I feeling?" I then answer, "I am feeling _____." Within a few minutes, any pain disappears.

The more dedicated you are right now to making this your new way of processing emotions, the faster you will develop a new unconscious process that keeps you permanently pain-free.

Is There A Best Time To Heal My Pain With the *Zero Pain Now* Process?

The best time to heal your pain is any time that you make the decision to dismiss the failed structural diagnosis that you have been using to manage your symptoms. Your healing starts with a decision to stop managing pain and use this process to heal, permanently. When you understand and believe that the cause of your pain is DPS, your symptoms will disappear.

Is A Hard Mattress Or A Soft Mattress Better For My Back?

Since your DPS pain has nothing to do with the anatomy of your back, no mattress will have any effect on your pain. The cure is to focus on your emotions, not on your mattress. Pick the mattress with which you're most comfortable.

Your unconscious mind is extremely busy while you sleep. That's when you dream. Some of my clients experience increased pain while sleeping, and also when they wake up. The brain's coincidence detector can link the pain to laying on a mattress and establish the mattress as the cause. This belief is incorrect. It's the unconscious emotions causing the problem. If this has been your problem, I suggest that you do an extra fifteen minutes of journaling about your emotions just before bedtime.

Should I Be Careful About How I Lift Things?

Remember that the cause of your pain and other symptoms is a psycho-physical disorder. It's not structural. There is no factual evidence that bending your knees to pick something up has any effect on your pain. A United States Post Office study in 1997 showed that "proper" lifting had absolutely no benefit whatsoever. I advise my clients that if you can comfortably pick up an item, do so. If it's too heavy, ask for help.

What About Fibromyalgia?

Fibromyalgia is Diversion Pain Syndrome. Follow the program exactly as written and you should rapidly heal your fibromyalgia symptoms.

Since My Personality Traits Are Common For DPS Sufferers, Do I Need To Change My Personality?

Every personality trait is beneficial in some context. There are great benefits in being a perfectionist. Many of the most successful people are perfectionists. What would the world be like without do gooders? All the traits I mentioned in the book can be wonderful. As you continue to use the techniques taught to you in this book you will develop a new strategy for your emotions. You don't need to change your personality. Simply acknowledge your negative emotions and you'll be fine.

Is It Possible For Me To Have DPS And Still Injure My Back?

It is possible to have an acute injury to your body. You can certainly strain a muscle when you do something extraordinary. An injury like this typically dissipates after a few days. The pain and symptoms that result from DPS are ongoing, recurrent, and repetitive, and last longer than a few days. Follow the program exactly as written and you will rapidly rid yourself of the pain and other symptoms.

Should I Continue To See My Medical Doctor Who Has Been Treating Me For These Problems?

Absolutely. Tell your medical doctor exactly what you are doing to heal your pain. Many cutting-edge doctors refer their patients with pain to me, and since the process works so well to heal pain, they are embracing this method.

I want to hear from you.

Follow us on:

www.facebook.com/adamhellersfanpage
Twitter: @adamheller

Send us your success stories.
success@zeropainnow.com

For more information go to:
www.zeropainnow.com

ACKNOWLEDGEMENTS

Writing this book has been a journey that would have been impossible without all my teachers, very close friends, and my family.

My good friend, and editor, Jahn Sanders-Levitt, brought patience, clarity, insight and professionalism to the project. I couldn't have written this book without her help.

Thank you to my close friend Chris Mitchell, who pushed me to write a book, and make the process available to the public.

Dr. John Sarno, was the pioneer who discovered the psychological cause of back and body pain. Without his years of research, this book and the *Zero Pain Now* Process would have been an impossibility.

Thank you to Howard Stern for discussing Dr. Sarno's work on his radio program. Howard's exuberance describing the process of how he cured his own pain, led me to begin my years of research, culminating in this book, and to the *Zero Pain Now* Process that has helped so many people eliminate their suffering physical pain.

Thank you to Dr. Tad James for creating and teaching me a critical portion of this process. Tad's training has been so useful for me to make positive personal changes, as well as help my clients.

Dr. Boris Borazjani, M.D., M.P.H. Long before this process was perfected, Boris understood Diversion Pain Syndrome, and envisioned all the ways this process will help people eliminate suffering. He lent me his name and his reputation. For that I will be eternally grateful.

Thank you to Dr. Eugene Levin M.D. F.A.C.P. Gene's sixty-two years practicing medicine and deep understanding and love of treating psychosomatic illness lend credibility to this book.

My mother, Carol, has always been my biggest supporter. Regardless of my age, she is still there for me. May she stay healthy and vibrant for many more years. I need her.

Thank you to my father, Lionel, may he rest in peace. Most of what I've learned about charity and service above self, I learned from him. He truly made the world a better place. I think of him, and smile, every day.

My son, Alton. I love every minute we are together. Whatever Alton chooses as his path in life, he will certainly make a huge difference.

My stepdaughter, Mirelle. I am looking forward to watching her flourish, and transform the world.

Thank you to Matt Hanover. Wow. Matt and I have been close friends for forty-five years. He trusted me, and this process, enough to cure his own debilitating shoulder pain that had been blamed on a torn rotator cuff. While the results of the *Zero Pain Now* Process were astounding, getting the message out has been a challenge and Matt has helped tremendously with that effort. Additional thanks to Soomi Rho, Lauren Sarafan, Grace Hawthorne, Lauren Levine, Dr. Marilee Friedrich, Kevin Stein, Paul Harris, and Liz Heller.

Thanks to my wife, Tamara. Little did she know when she moved to Laguna Beach from Toronto to marry me, the sacrifices she would make. She has placed many of her dreams on hold so I can reach mine. She continues to inspire me and support me through this process.

It may be cliche but, **I AM THE LUCKIEST MAN IN THE WORLD**!

ABOUT THE AUTHOR

Adam Heller has helped thousands of people rapidly solve problems. He spent a decade helping his clients heal from a divorce, the loss of a loved one, lose weight, and overcome fears, phobias and panic attacks. Adam has developed new techniques that empower people to change their behaviors to overcome problems, and produce success.

Three years ago Adam began examining the link between physical pain and emotions. He expanded on a rich body of evidence supporting the theory of what he came to name Diversion Pain Syndrome. The investigation produced the method that Adam titled *Zero Pain Now* Process. Most of Adam's time is now spent teaching people how to heal their own physical pain.

Adam is the originator of Adam Heller's *Zero Pain Now* Process and Rapid Life Change. He is a Certified Instructor of Neuro Linguistic Programming (NLP), and a Certified Master in Integrative Coaching, Time Line Therapy™, Hypnosis and Spiritual Divorce. Adam is a sought after keynote speaker, and a frequent subject for interviews across all media.

INDEX

S

Sadness 150, 194, 211
Sanders-Levitt, Jahn 218
Sanders, Tony 198
Sarno, John 23, 34, 40, 43, 47, 65, 66, 67, 160, 218
Scoliosis 148, 158
Shame 150, 194, 211
Simon, David 35
Smith, Cheryl 128
Spinal Stenosis 148
Spiritual 35, 110, 151, 167, 195, 211, 221

T

Tendonitis 69
Tension Myositis Syndrome 47, 66
Time Line Therapy 40, 221
TMJ 69, 148, 172

U

Unconscious Mind 87, 123, 132, 147, 149, 150, 151, 154, 157, 158, 170, 172, 174, 182, 203, 204, 208, 209, 214

W

Whiplash Syndrome 69, 116, 117, 168

X

X-Ray 17, 63, 65, 70, 79, 111, 119, 148, 158, 160, 163

CPSIA information can be obtained at www.ICGtesting.com
Printed in the USA
LVOW04s2230171014

409307LV00025B/796/P